Detox Cookbook for Anyone

Get Rid of Those Toxins in Your Body in An Easy Way

BY: Valeria Ray

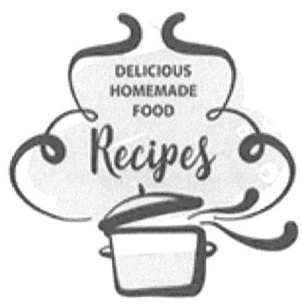

License Notes

A Special Reward for Purchasing My Book!

Thank you, cherished reader, for purchasing my book and taking the time to read it. As a special reward for your decision, I would like to offer a gift of free and discounted books directly to your inbox. All you need to do is fill in the box below with your email address and name to start getting amazing offers in the comfort of your own home. You will never miss an offer because a reminder will be sent to you. Never miss a deal and get great deals without having to leave the house! Subscribe now and start saving!

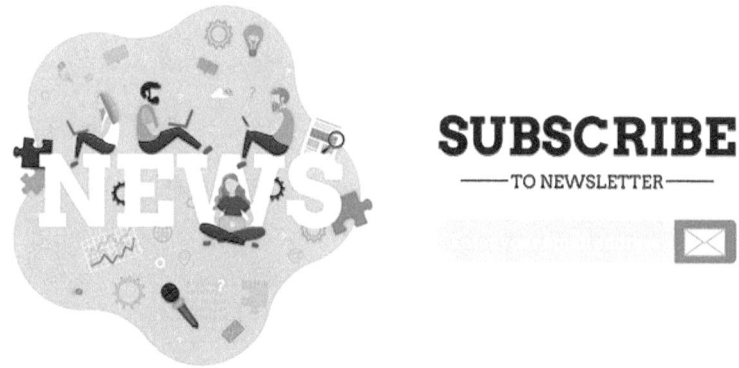

https://valeria-ray.gr8.com

Contents

Chapter I - Detox Recipes

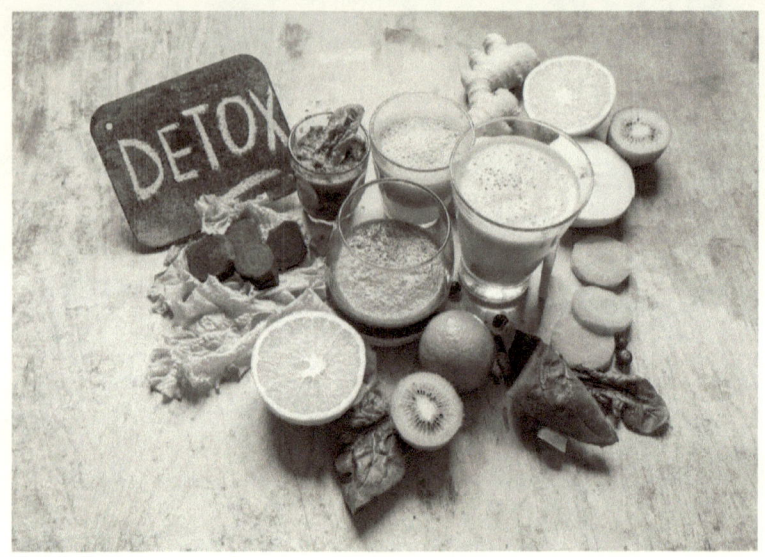

MMMMMMMMMMMMMMMMMMMMMMMMMMMMMMMM

(1) Ginger, Pear, Cinnamon Vanilla Bean Infused Water

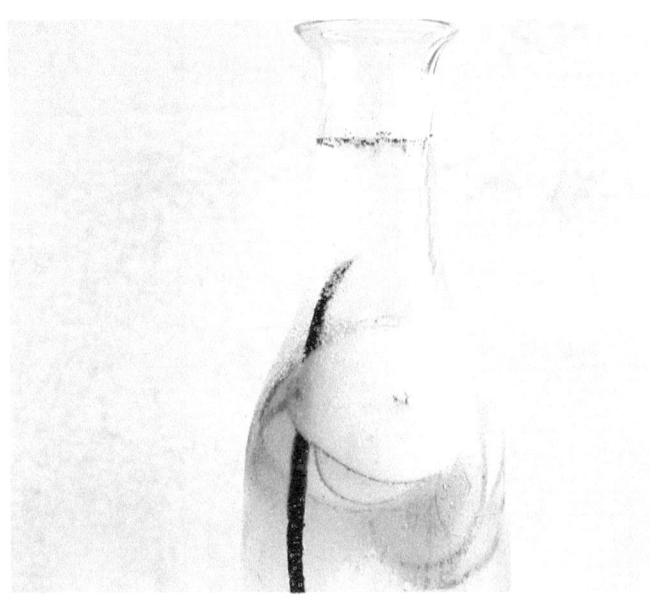

A detox drink doesn't have to be yucky. Here is a tasty drink that will aid in cleansing your body of unwanted toxins.

Yield: 48 Fl. oz.

Preparation Time: 5 minutes + chilling time

List of Ingredients:

- 5 sliced pears
- ½ knob ginger, thinly sliced
- 1 c. ice
- 1 teaspoon cinnamon powder
- 1 vanilla bean
- 6 c. water

MMMMMMMMMMMMMMMMMMMMMMMMMMMMMMMM

Methods:

1. Add your pears, ginger, and vanilla bean in a large pitcher.

2. Add in your cinnamon, top with ice cubes and pour in the water.

3. Cover and allow to chill for a minimum of 2 hours or overnight.

4. Serve and Enjoy!

(2) Lemon, Mint Cucumber Infused Water

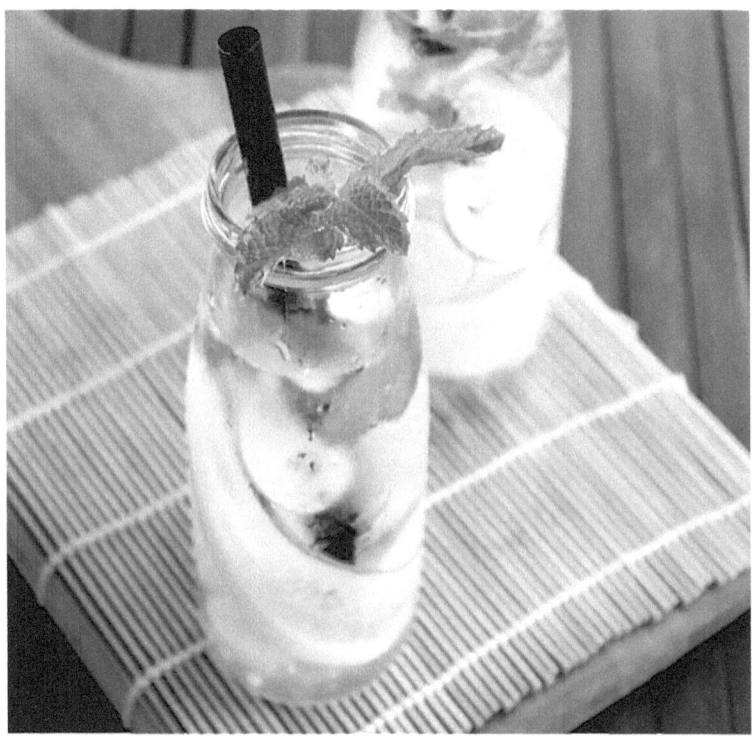

This detox mix is perfect for flushing our bodies of unwanted fat.

Yield: 48 Fl. oz.

Preparation Time: 5 minutes + chilling time

List of Ingredients:

- 6 c. water
- 1 c. mint leaves
- 1 sliced orange
- ½ c. cucumber slices

MMMMMMMMMMMMMMMMMMMMMMMMMMMMMMMM

Methods:

1. Combine all the Ingredients in a pitcher.

2. Refrigerate for 2 hours or overnight.

3. Serve in the morning and drink through the day.

(3) Flush Cleanse Water

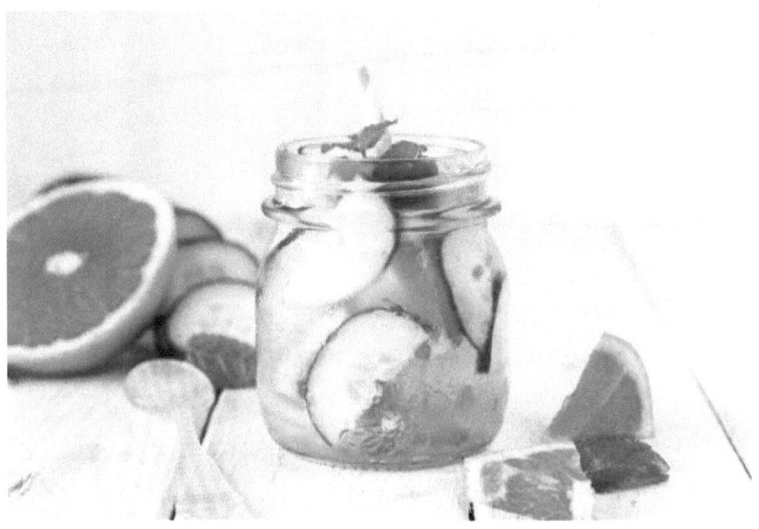

This detox mix helps to naturally flush your body. It is a simple recipe to prepare with a lot of health benefits.

Makes: 48 Fl. oz.

Preparation Time: 5 minutes + chilling time

List of Ingredients:

- ½ gallon Water
- 6 Pink Grapefruits, cut into wedges
- 1 sliced Tangerine
- ½ sliced Cucumber
- 2 Mint leaves
- 1 c. Ice

MMMMMMMMMMMMMMMMMMMMMMMMMMMMMMM

Methods:

1. Combine all the Ingredients in a pitcher.

2. Refrigerate for 2 hours or overnight.

3. Serve in the morning and drink through the day.

(4) Black Charcoal Lemonade

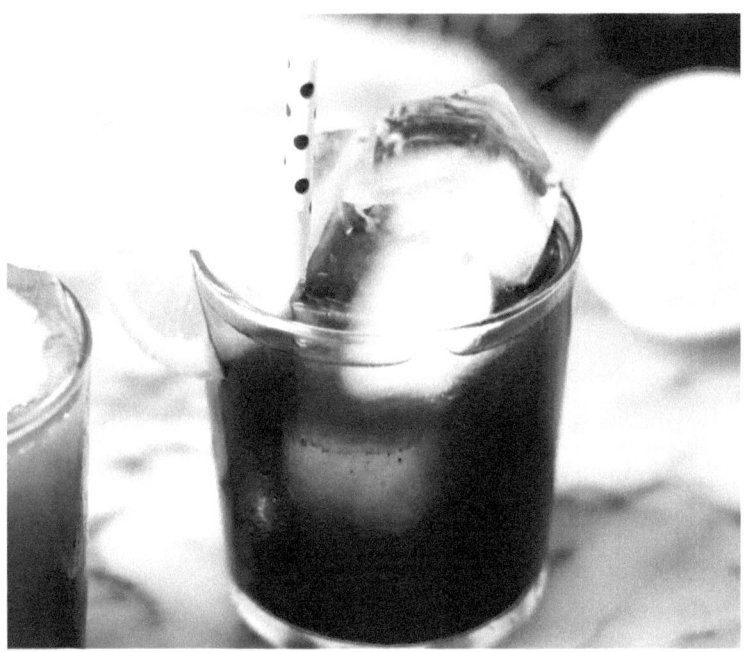

This drink may look unappealing but it surprisingly tastes just like regular lemonade. Charcoal has been said to help relieve the body of unwanted gases and can be purchased in tablets from a local pharmacy.

Yield: 1

Preparation Time: 5 minutes

List of Ingredients:

- 4 c. filtered Water
- ¼ c. Lemon Juice
- 15 drops Stevia
- 1 capsule activated Charcoal

MMMMMMMMMMMMMMMMMMMMMMMMMMMMMMMM

Methods:

1.   In   a   mixing   bowl,   bring   all   the above Ingredients together and mix.

2. Serve over ice, enjoy.

(5) Cucumber, Strawberry Thyme Infused Water

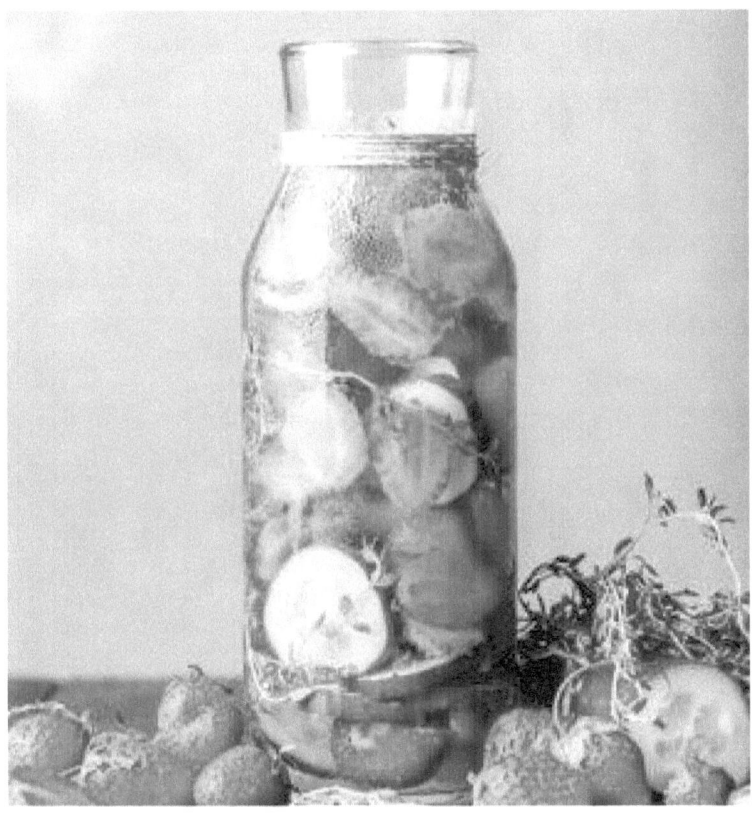

Here is a drink that provides a light and refreshing cleanse for your body.

Yield: 48 Fl. oz.

Preparation Time: 5 minutes + chilling time

List of Ingredients:

- 1-pint sliced strawberries
- 6 small sprigs lemon thyme
- 1 sliced cucumber
- 6 c. water

MMMMMMMMMMMMMMMMMMMMMMMMMMMMMMMM

Methods:

1. Bruise the thyme and place into a pitcher.

2. Add the sliced strawberries, and cucumber.

3. Add water to the pitcher until full and place in the refrigerator for 2 hours or overnight.

4. Serve after.

(6) Immune-Boosting Strawberry Smoothie

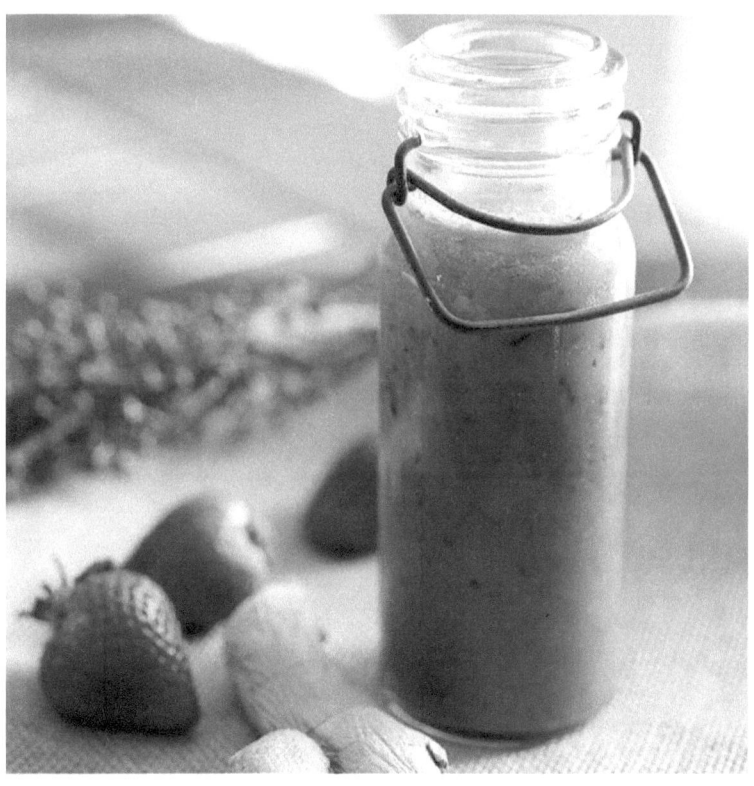

Eliminate processed sugar from your body, and introduce nutrients such as fiber, potassium, and vitamin C with this detox smoothie.

Yield: 1

Preparation Time: 10 minutes

List of Ingredients:

- ½ frozen Banana
- 1 c. frozen Strawberries
- ½ frozen Beets
- ½ teaspoons Ginger, grated
- 1 c. Coconut Milk
- ½ teaspoons Lime Juice
- 4 Ice Cubes
- 1 handful Spinach

MMMMMMMMMMMMMMMMMMMMMMMMMMMMMMMM

Methods:

1. In a blender, mix all Ingredients and pulse until smooth.

2. Serve, and enjoy.

(7) Blueberry, Lime Cilantro Infused Water

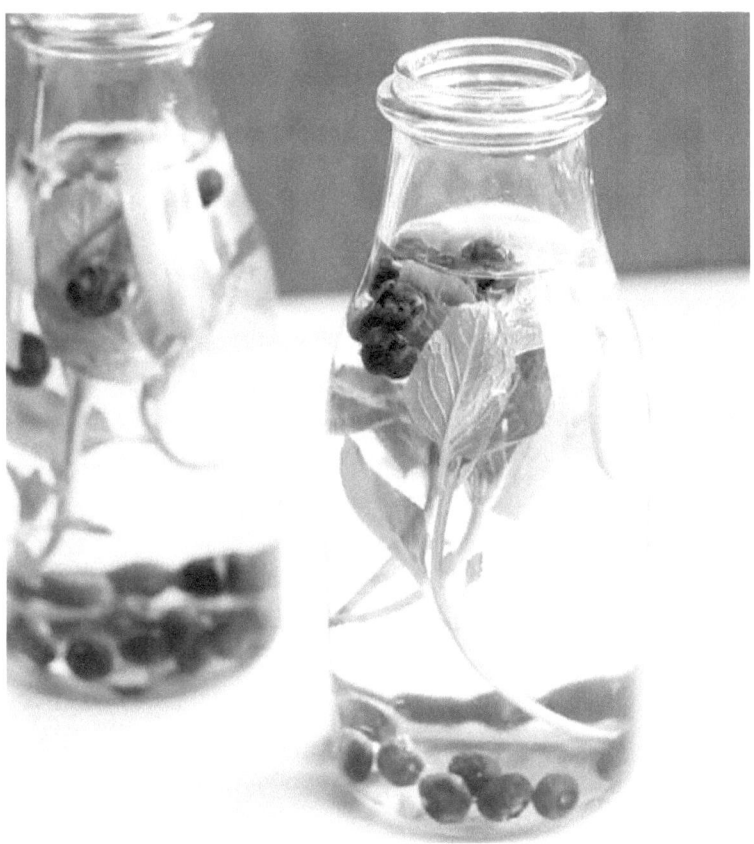

This mix provides a unique combination of sweet, tangy and just enough acidity to give it the edge it needs to be delicious.

Yield: 48 Fl. oz.

Preparation Time: 5 minutes + chilling time

List of Ingredients:

- 1-pint sliced blueberries
- 1 sliced lemon
- 1 small handful cilantro
- 6 c. water

MMMMMMMMMMMMMMMMMMMMMMMMMMMMMMMM

Methods:

1. In a pitcher, combine all the Ingredients.

2. Refrigerate for 3 hours before serving.

(8) Lemon Ginger Detox Drink

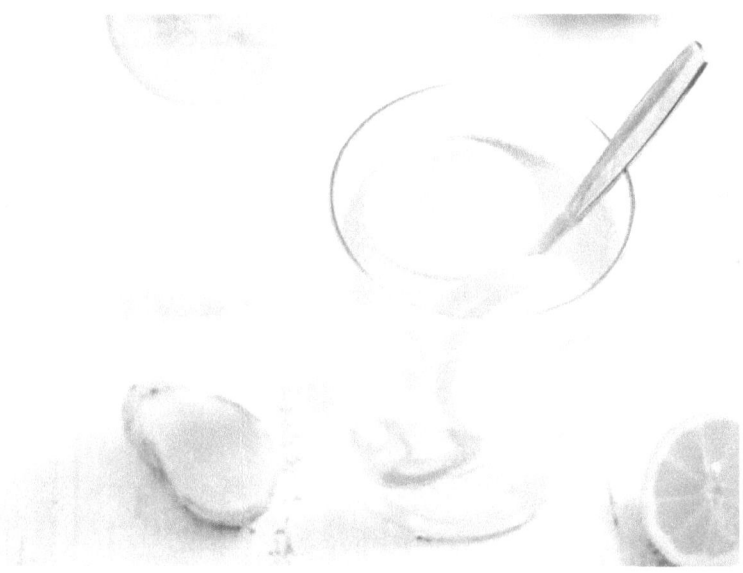

Here is a detox drink that helps to shed your body of unwanted fat.

Yield: 1

Preparation Time: 5 minutes

List of Ingredients:

- 12 oz. Water
- ½ Lemon Juiced
- ½ inch knob Ginger, grated

MMMMMMMMMMMMMMMMMMMMMMMMMMMMMMMMMM

Methods:

1. Use a large bowl to mix together all Ingredients.

2. Serve over ice, enjoy.

(9) Raspberry, Kiwi Peach Infused Water

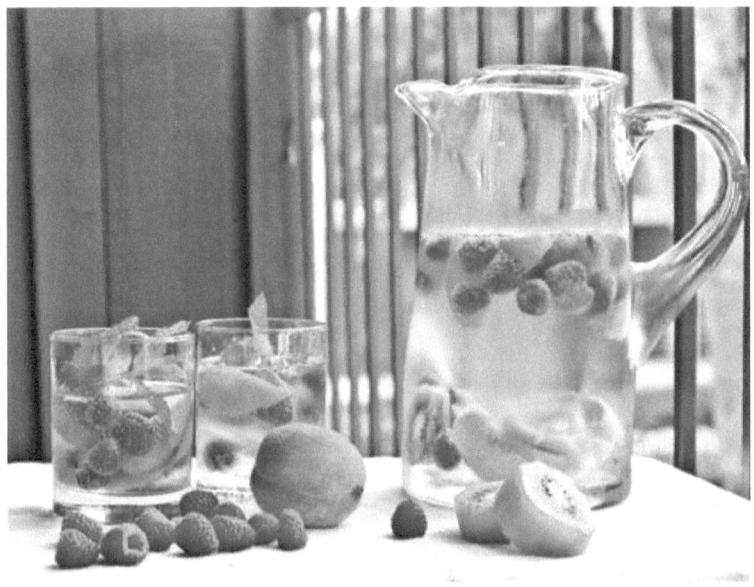

This mix is perfect for working out those hot summer days.

Yield: 48 Fl. Oz.

Preparation Time: 5 minutes + chilling time

List of Ingredients:

- 5 peach slices, frozen
- 7 sliced kiwis, frozen
- 1-pint raspberries
- 1 sprig mint
- 1 c. ice
- 3 c. water

MMMMMMMMMMMMMMMMMMMMMMMMMMMMMM

Methods:

1. Drop the peaches, kiwi, and raspberries in a large pitcher.

2. Cover with ice and add water.

3. Refrigerate for 4 hours before serving.

4. Drink through the day.

(10) Peppermint Tea

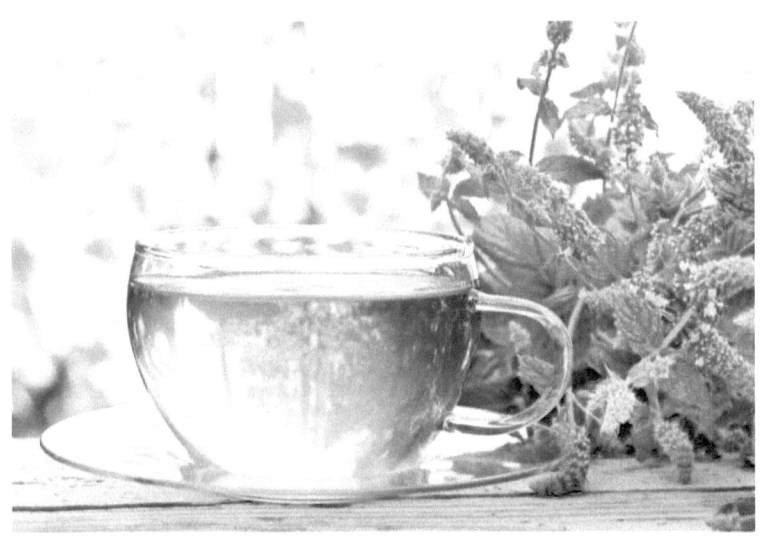

This herbal tea can help in your detox to help with abdominal gas and bloat.

Preparation Time: 37 minutes

Yield: 4

List of Ingredients:

- ½ c. Peppermint Leaf, dried
- 4 c. Water, hot

MMMMMMMMMMMMMMMMMMMMMMMMMMMMMMMMM

Methods:

1. Set your water on to boil. Once boiling, add in your peppermint leaves and remove from heat.

2. Allow to sit for 5 minutes while covered.

3. Strain, serve and enjoy

(11) Rose, Lemon Strawberry Infused Water

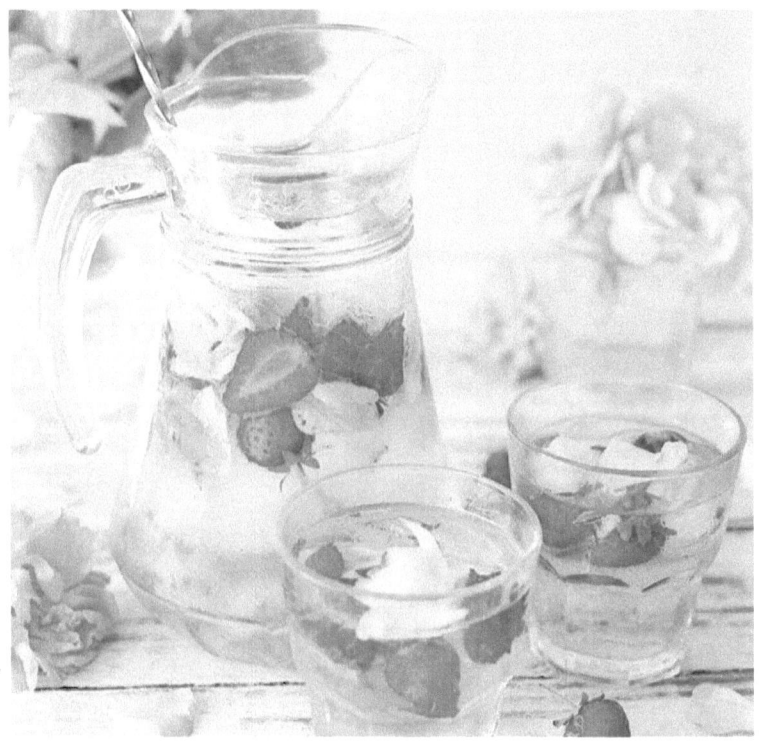

This mix uses the common rose and other easily available Ingredients to help cleanse your body.

Yield: 48 Fl. oz.

Preparation Time: 5 minutes + chilling time

List of Ingredients:

- 1 c. strawberries
- 1 tablespoon rose petals, dried
- 1 sliced lemon
- 6 c. water

MMMMMMMMMMMMMMMMMMMMMMMMMMMMMMMM

Methods:

1. Place the strawberries, rose petals and lemon in a pitcher.

2. Pour in water and muddle gently.

3. Refrigerate for 24 hours.

4. Strain through the sieve and discard the solids.

5. Serve after.

(12) Ginger Tea

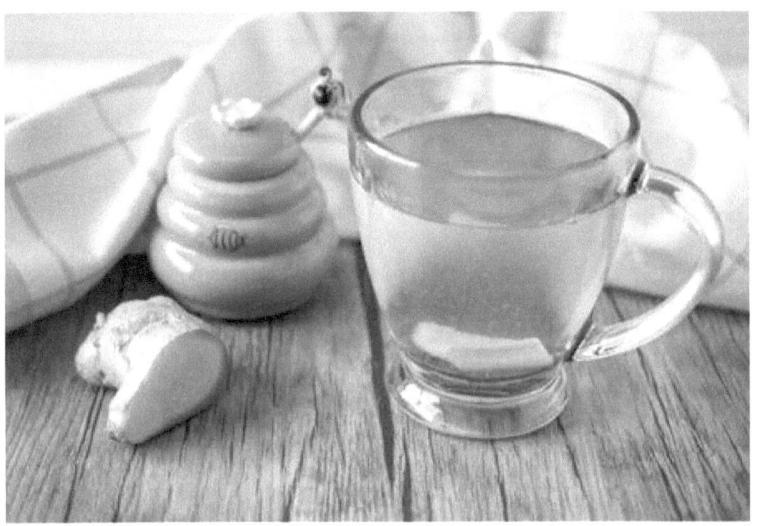

This is a classic detox tea that has been known to help curb an upset stomach, nausea and even subdue vomiting.

Preparation Time: 15 minutes

Yield: 2

List of Ingredients:

- 3 teaspoons. Gingerroot, grated
- 3 c. Boiling Water

MMMMMMMMMMMMMMMMMMMMMMMMMMMMMMMM

Methods:

1. Combine your Ingredients together and allow to rest, covered for at least 10 minutes.

2. Serve and Enjoy!

(13) Grapefruit Pineapple Infused Water

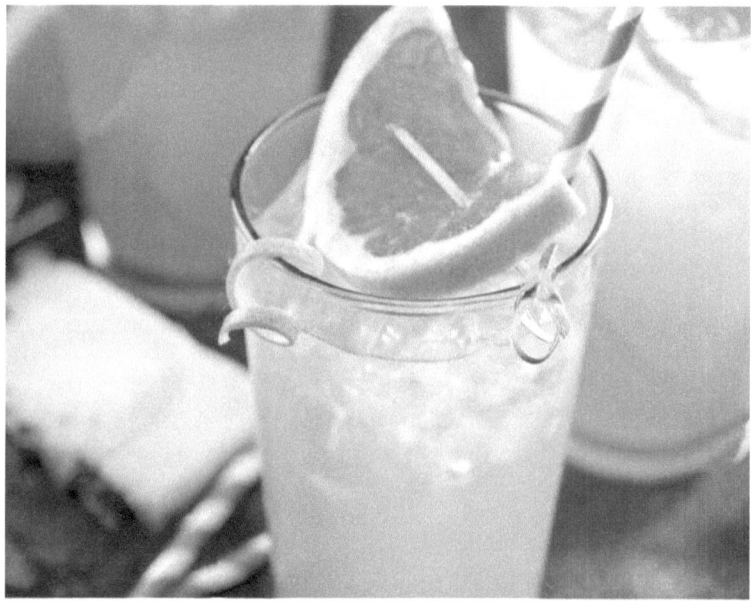

This tropical blend offers deliciousness while promoting weight loss and proper blood circulation.

Yield: 64 Fl. oz.

Preparation Time: 5 minutes + chilling time

List of Ingredients:

- ½ c. peeled and thinly sliced pineapple
- 1 thinly sliced grapefruit
- 2 c. ice
- 6 c. Water

MMMMMMMMMMMMMMMMMMMMMMMMMMMMMMMMM

Methods:

1. In a large pitcher, combine the pineapple and orange.

2. Top with ice.

3. Pour in water to the top and cover.

4. Refrigerate for 1 hour before serving.

(14) Red Apple and Carrot Tea

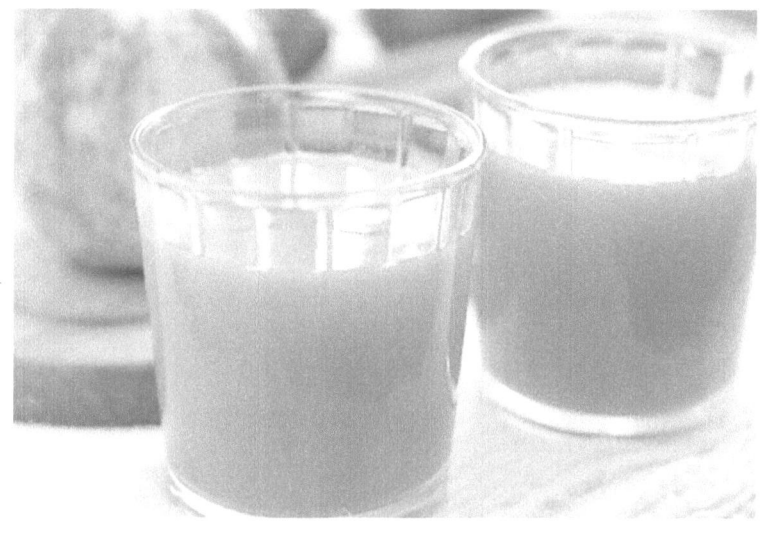

This detox tea is known to help cure chronic constipation.

Preparation Time: 6 minutes

Yield: 3

List of Ingredients:

- 1 c. peeled red apples, chunks
- 2 sliced carrots
- ½ c. seeded lychee
- 2 c. water

MMMMMMMMMMMMMMMMMMMMMMMMMMMMMMMM

Methods:

1. Blend apples with carrots, lychee, and water.

2. Using a saucepan, place in all the Ingredients and allow to come to a boil.

3. Kill the heat and allow to sit for 5 minutes.

4. Strain, serve and enjoy!

(15) Strawberry, Lime Mint Infused Water

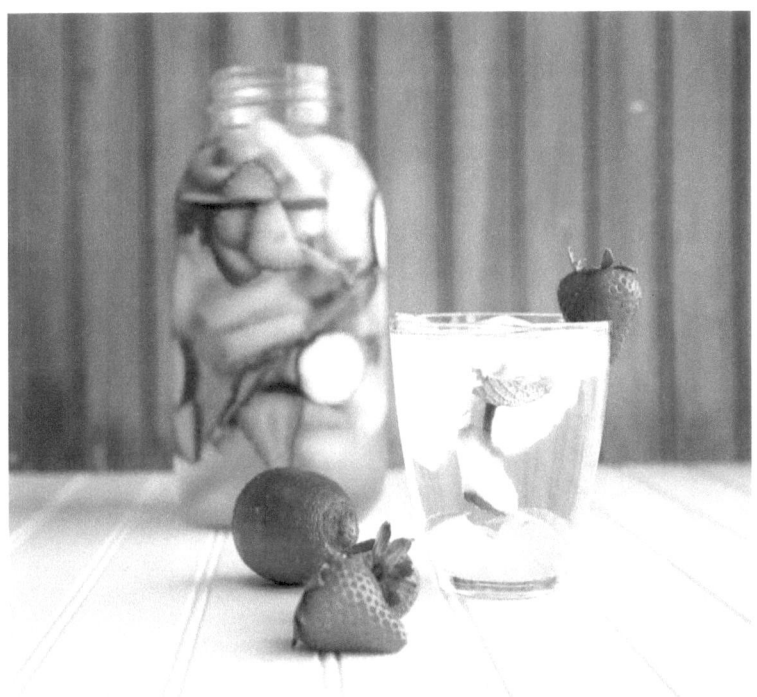

Boost your metabolism, while jazzing up your day with this tasty detox recipe.

Yield: 48 Fl. oz.

Preparation Time: 5 minutes + chilling time

List of Ingredients:

- 6 c. water
- 1-pint sliced strawberries
- 3 sliced limes
- 10 mint leaves

MMMMMMMMMMMMMMMMMMMMMMMMMMMMMMM

Methods:

1. Combine all the Ingredients in a pitcher.

2. Refrigerate for 2 hours or overnight.

3. Serve in the morning and drink through the day.

(16) Rooibos Tea

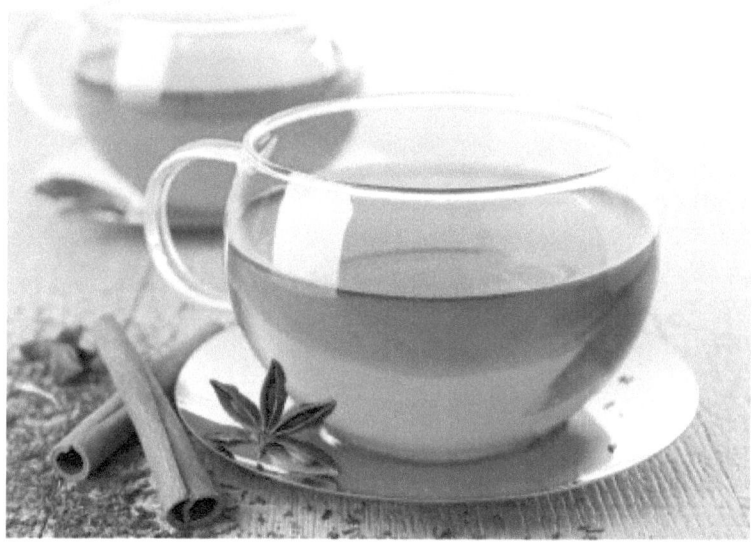

This detox drink is packed with vitamin C, as well as other antioxidants and minerals.

Preparation Time: 30 minutes

Yield: 4

List of Ingredients:

- ½ c. Rooibos
- 4 c. Water, hot

MMMMMMMMMMMMMMMMMMMMMMMMMMMMMMMM

Methods:

1. Set your water on to boil. Once boiling, add in your rooibos pieces and remove from heat.

2. Allow to sit for 15 minutes while covered.

3. Strain, serve and enjoy

(17) Pink Grapefruit Cucumber Infused Water

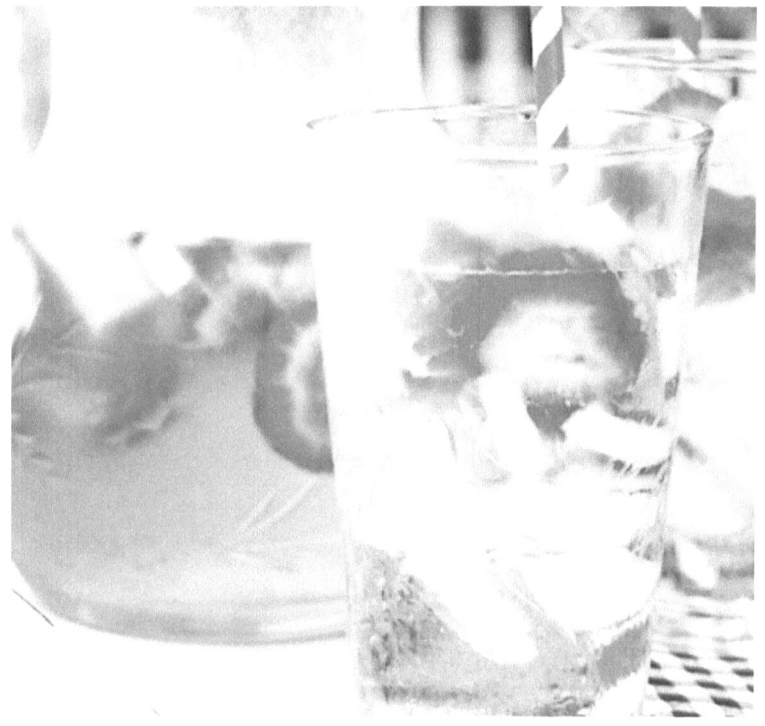

This detox mix helps with weight loss alongside other benefits to the body.

Yield: 48 Fl. oz.

Preparation Time: 5 minutes + chilling time

List of Ingredients:

- 6 c. water
- 2 sliced pink grapefruits
- ½ c. cucumber slices

MMMMMMMMMMMMMMMMMMMMMMMMMMMMMMMM

Methods:

1. Combine all the Ingredients in a pitcher.

2. Refrigerate for 2 hours or overnight.

3. Serve in the morning and drink through the day.

(18) Chamomile Tea

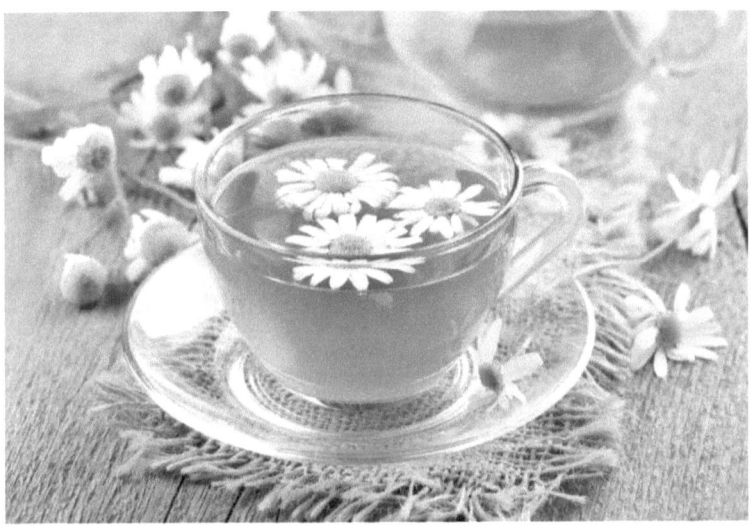

The herbal detox tea is said to aid in the digestion process which makes it a brilliant option during a detox.

Preparation Time: 10 minutes

Yield: 2

List of Ingredients:

- 2 tablespoons Chamomile Flowers
- 2 c. Water

MMMMMMMMMMMMMMMMMMMMMMMMMMMMMMMMMM

Methods:

1. Set your water on to boil. Once boiling, add in your chamomile and remove from heat.

2. Allow to sit for 5 minutes while covered.

3. Strain, serve and enjoy

(19) Lemony Mint Water

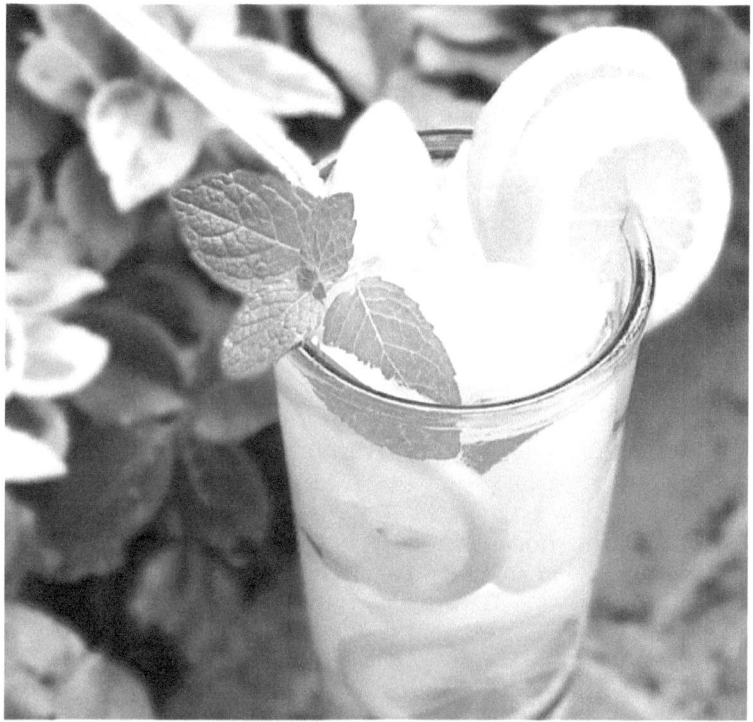

Kick start your metabolism with this morning detox water.

Yield: 48 Fl. oz.

Preparation Time: 5 minutes + chilling time

List of Ingredients:

- 6 c. water
- 1 c. mint leaves
- 3 sliced lemons

MMMMMMMMMMMMMMMMMMMMMMMMMMMMMMMM

Methods:

1. Combine all the Ingredients in a pitcher.

2. Refrigerate for 2 hours or overnight.

3. Serve in the morning and drink through the day.

(20) Lemon Balm Tea

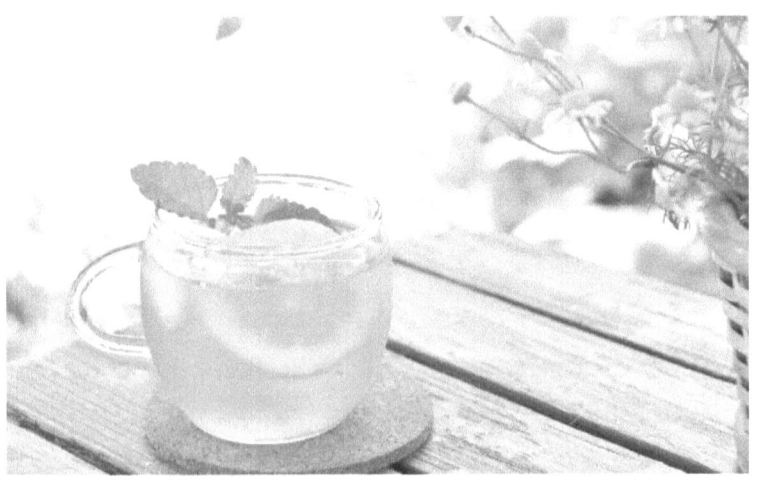

This detox tea is great for relaxation as it helps to relieve the body of stress hormones.

Preparation Time: 20 minutes

Yield: 4

List of Ingredients:

- 1 c. Lemon Balm
- 5 c. Water
- 1 tablespoon Lemon Zest

MMMMMMMMMMMMMMMMMMMMMMMMMMMMMMMM

Methods:

1. Set your water on to boil. Once boiling add in your lemon balm, and zest then remove from heat.

2. Allow to sit for 10 mutes while covered.

3. Strain, serve and enjoy

(21) Pineapple, Orange Ginger Infused Water

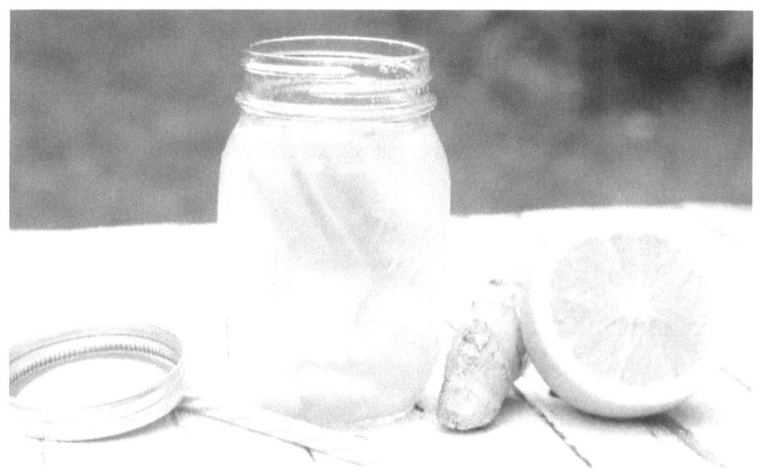

This mix is perfect for flushing our bodies of unwanted toxins.

Yield: 48 Fl. oz.

Preparation Time: 5 minutes + chilling time

List of Ingredients:

- 6 c. water
- 1 sliced pineapple
- 1 sliced orange
- ½ c. ginger slices

MMMMMMMMMMMMMMMMMMMMMMMMMMMMMMMM

Methods:

1. Combine all the above Ingredients in a pitcher.

2. Refrigerate for 2 hours or overnight.

3. Serve in the morning and drink through the day.

(22) Dandelion Tea

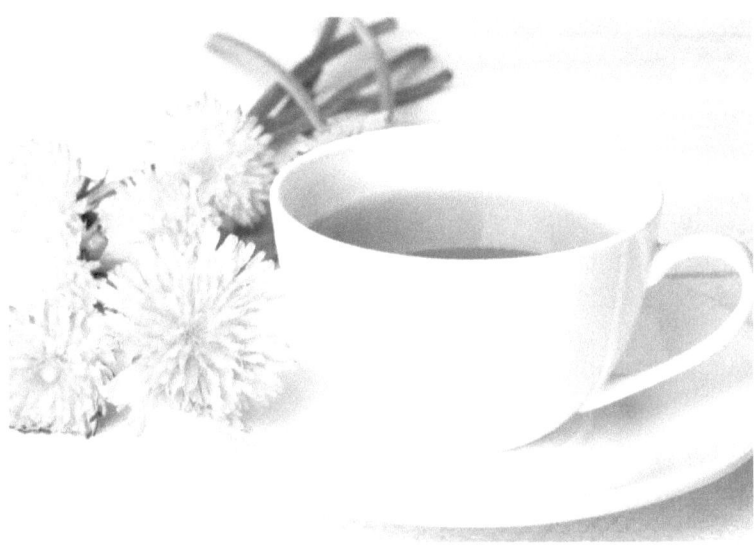

This detox tea works to cleanse your livers, and aids in bile production which is vital in the digestion process.

Preparation Time: 10 minutes

Yield: 2

List of Ingredients:

- 2 tablespoons Dandelion Flowers
- 2 c. Water

MMMMMMMMMMMMMMMMMMMMMMMMMMMMMMMMMMMM

Methods:

1. Set your water on to boil. Once boiling, add in your dandelion and remove from heat.

2. Allow to sit for 5 minutes while covered.

3. Strain, serve and enjoy

(23) Mango Ginger Water

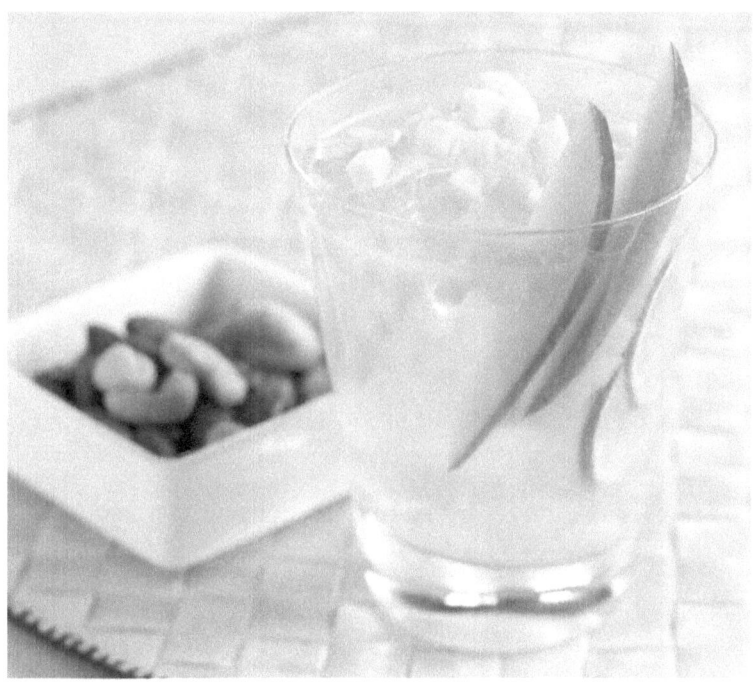

This detox water will keep you refreshed while detoxifying the body.

Yield: 64 Fl. oz.

Preparation Time: 5 minutes + inactive time

List of Ingredients:

- 1 c. diced mango
- 1-inch ginger, peeled and sliced
- 2 c. ice
- Water, to top off

MMMMMMMMMMMMMMMMMMMMMMMMMMMMMMMM

Methods:

1. Peel and slice the ginger in 3-4-coin size slices.

2. Transfer the ginger into a pitcher along with mango.

3. Top with 2 cups ice and fill with water.

4. Refrigerate for 3 hours.

5. Serve after.

(24) Hibiscus Tea

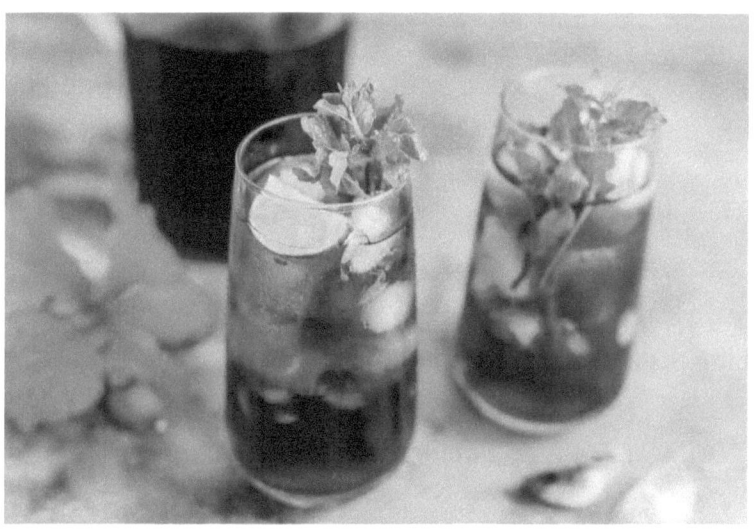

This detox tea is said to keep high cholesterol and high blood pressure at bay.

Preparation Time: 10 minutes

Yield: 2

List of Ingredients:

- 4 tablespoons Hibiscus Flowers
- 2 c. Water

MMMMMMMMMMMMMMMMMMMMMMMMMMMMMMM

Methods:

1. Set your water on to boil. Once boiling, add in your hibiscus and remove from heat.

2. Allow to sit for 5 minutes while covered.

3. Strain, serve and enjoy

(25) Citrus Mint Infused Water

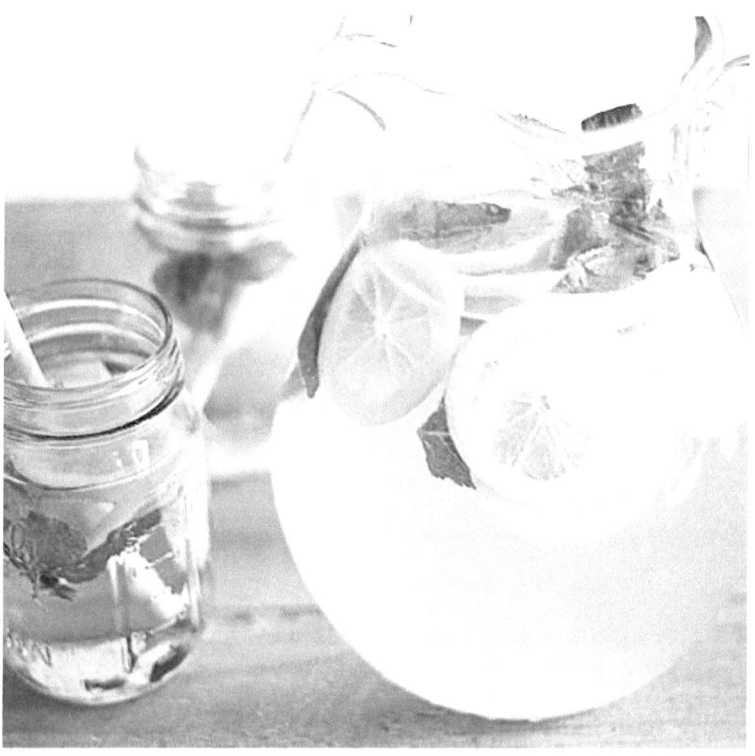

Here is a delicious detox water that helps to promote weight loss.

Yield: 64 Fl. oz.

Preparation Time: 5 minutes + chilling time

List of Ingredients:

- ½ segmented red grapefruit
- 2 mint leaves
- ½ sliced lemon
- 1 sliced cucumber
- ½ sliced lime
- ½ gallon spring water

MMMMMMMMMMMMMMMMMMMMMMMMMMMMMMM

Methods:

1. Wash and prepare the Ingredients.

2. Place all the Ingredients in a pitcher.

3. Refrigerate for 2 hours.

4. Serve after.

(26) Green Tea

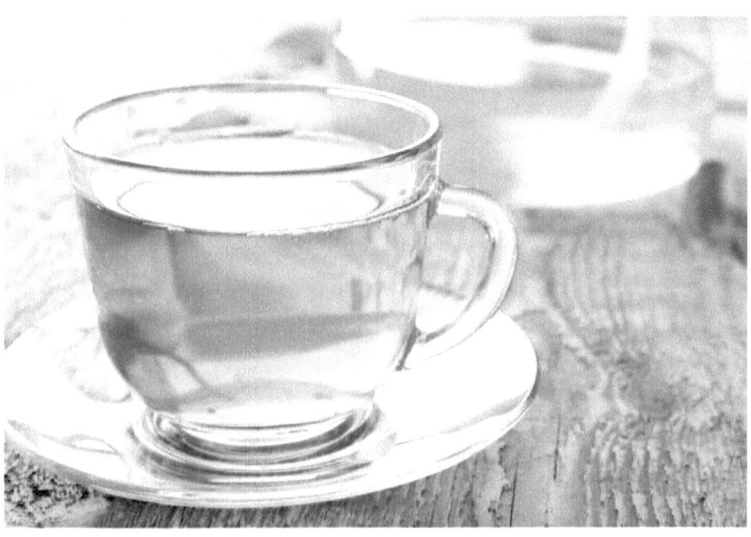

This detox tea carries a myriad of health benefits, including fat loss, improving brain function, and even lowering the risk of cancer.

Preparation Time: 20 minutes

Yield: 2

List of Ingredients:

- 4 tablespoons Camellia Sinensis Leaves, fresh
- 2 c. Water

MMMMMMMMMMMMMMMMMMMMMMMMMMMMMMMMMM

Methods:

1. Set your water on to boil. Once boiling, add in your Camellia and remove from heat.

2. Allow to sit for 10 mutes while covered.

3. Strain, serve and enjoy

(27) Pork Bone Broth

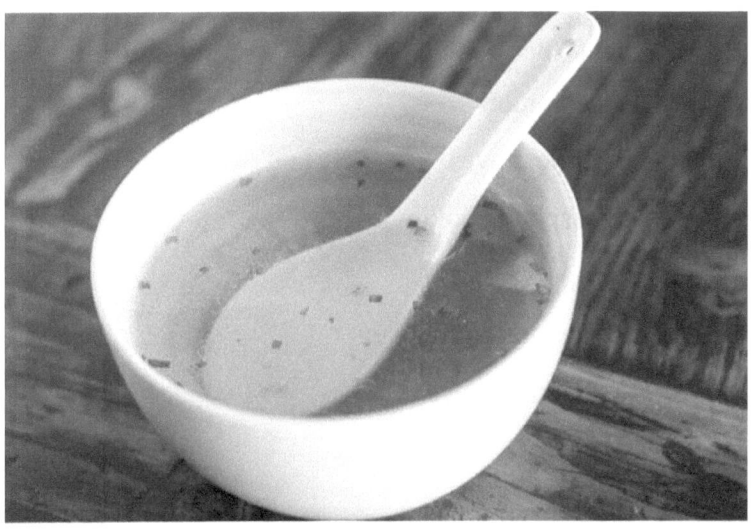

This highly nutritious delight is made with just a few and simple.

List of Ingredients:

Preparation Time: 2 hours

Yield: 5

List of Ingredients:

- 1 oz. cleaned pork bones
- 2 tablespoons apple cider vinegar
- 1 sliced onion
- 5-6 garlic cloves
- 1 tablespoon cooking oil
- ½ teaspoons salt
- ½ teaspoons white pepper
- 1-inch ginger slice
- 5 c. water

MMMMMMMMMMMMMMMMMMMMMMMMMMMMMMMM

Methods:

1. In a large skillet add bones with water, onion, garlic, ginger, oil, vinegar, salt, pepper, and stir. Cover with lid.

2. Change source of heat to low and cook for 2 hours.

3. Strain the broth and discard residue.

4. Serve hot and enjoy.

(28) Orange Carrot Lemon Ginger Tea

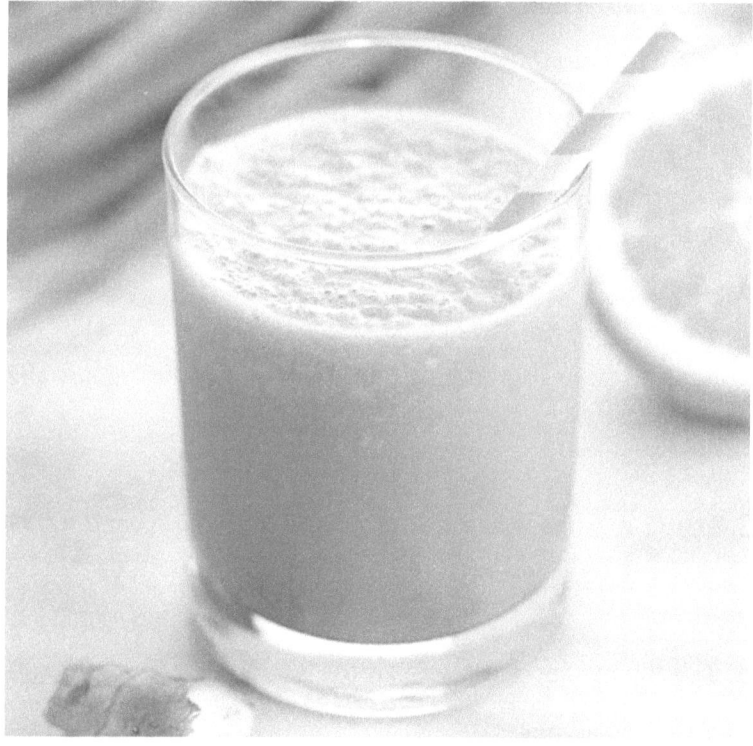

If you love strong citrusy drinks, then you will love this!

Yield: 5 cups

Preparation Time: 11 minutes

List of Ingredients:

- 4 halved Oranges, halved
- 12 oz. diced Carrots
- ½ inch knob Ginger, grated
- ½ Lemon juiced
- 4 c. Water

MMMMMMMMMMMMMMMMMMMMMMMMMMMMMMMM

Methods:

1. Pour all your Ingredients into the Vitamix and secure the lid.

2. Using a saucepan, place in all the Ingredients and allow to come to a boil.

3. Kill the heat and allow to sit for 5 minutes.

4. Strain, serve and enjoy!

(29) Chicken Bone Broth

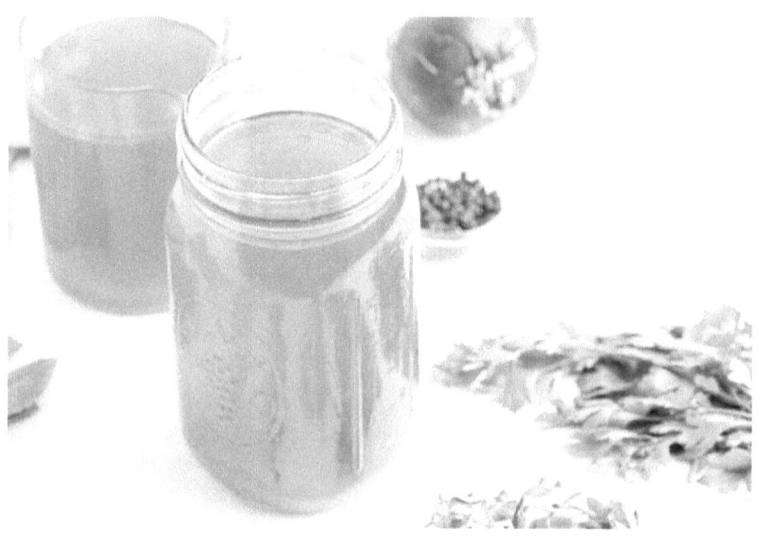

This broth is perfect for soothing stomach aches. It is delicious and easy to prepare.

Preparation Time: 2 hours

Yield: 5

List of Ingredients:

- 1 oz. cleaned chicken bones
- 2 tablespoons apple cider vinegar
- 1 sliced onion
- 5-6 garlic cloves
- 1 tablespoon cooking oil
- ½ teaspoons salt
- ½ teaspoons white pepper
- 1-inch ginger slice
- 5 c. water

MMMMMMMMMMMMMMMMMMMMMMMMMMMMMMMMM

Methods:

1. In a large skillet add bones with water, onion, garlic, ginger, oil, vinegar, salt, pepper, and stir. Cover with lid.

2. Set heat to low and let cook for 2 hours.

3. Strain the broth and discard residue.

4. Serve hot and enjoy.

(30) Lemon, Mint Cucumber Infused Water

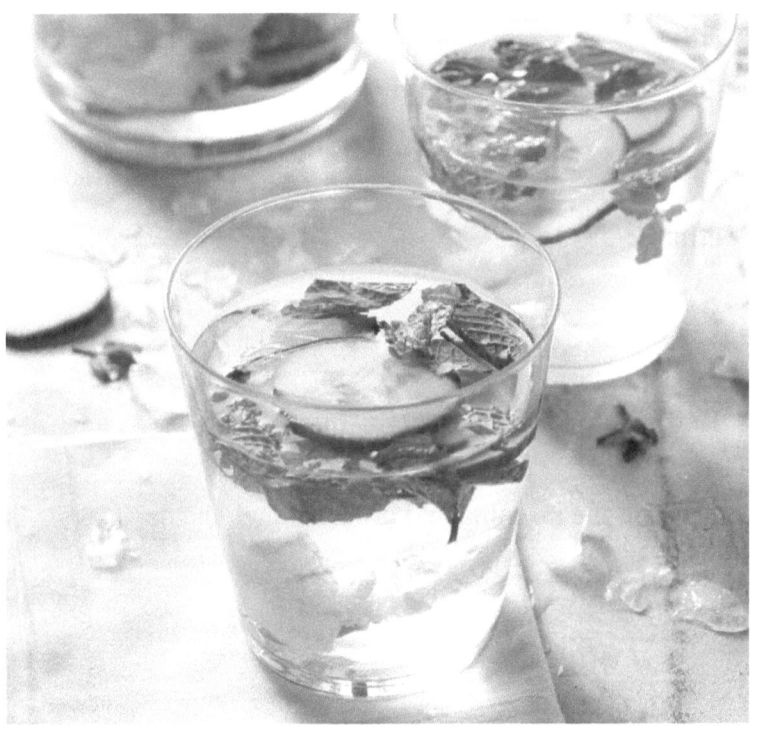

This detox mix is perfect for flushing our bodies of unwanted toxins.

Yield: 48 Fl. oz.

Preparation Time: 5 minutes + chilling time

List of Ingredients:

- 6 c. water
- 1 sliced grapefruit
- 1 sliced orange
- ½ c. cucumber slices

MMMMMMMMMMMMMMMMMMMMMMMMMMMMMMMMM

Methods:

1. Combine all the above Ingredients in a pitcher.

2. Refrigerate for 2 hours or overnight.

3. Serve in the morning and drink through the day.

Chapter II - Bonus Green Detox Recipes

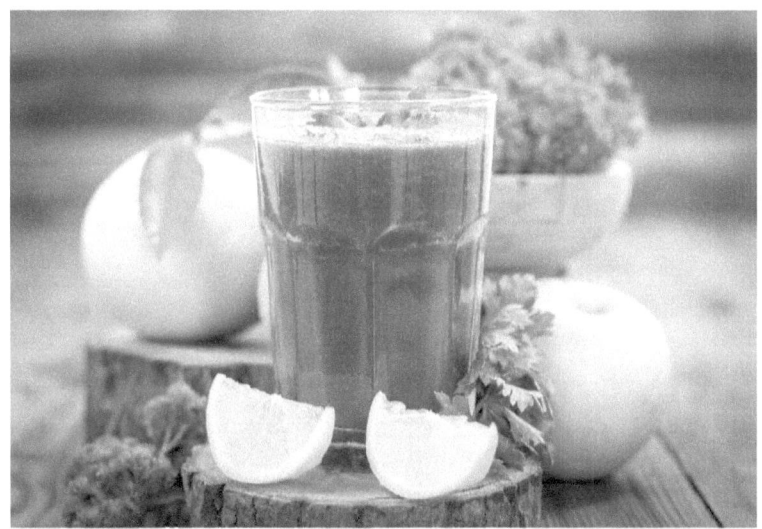

MMMMMMMMMMMMMMMMMMMMMMMMMMMMMMMM

(31) Berry Kale Creamy Green Smoothie

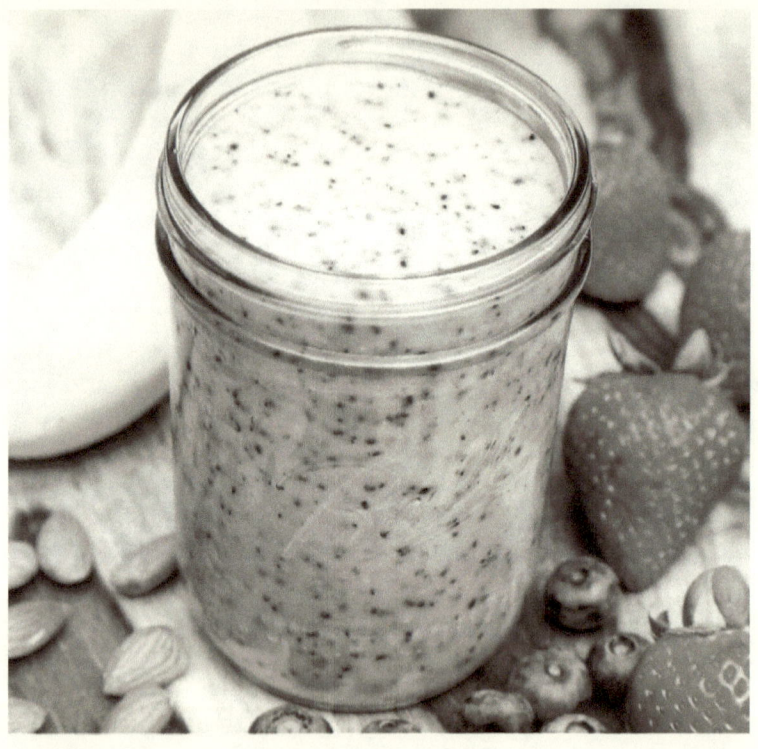

Assorted berries, bananas and Kale are a delicious combination sure to please.

Yield: 50 oz.

Preparation Time: 5 minutes

List of Ingredients:

- 2 frozen and peeled Bananas
- 2 c. Strawberries
- 1 c. Blueberries, frozen
- 6 pitted and chopped Dates
- 2 c. Water
- 1 large bunch Kale
- 2 tablespoons Flax Seeds

MMMMMMMMMMMMMMMMMMMMMMMMMMMMMMMM

Methods:

In a blender, add all Ingredients except for the greens and pulse a few times. Then add in the Greens and process on high until you have a smooth and creamy texture. Serve.

(32) Simple Green Smoothie

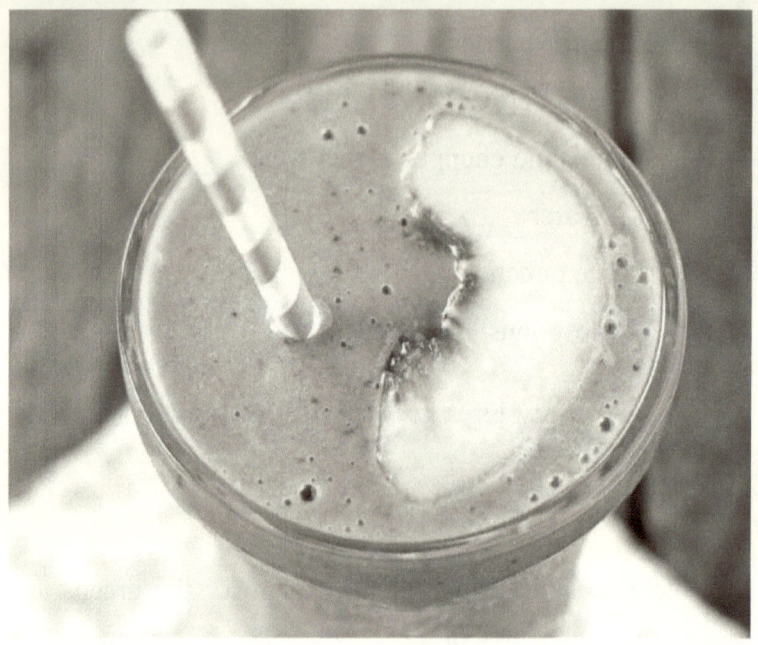

This is the easiest Green Smoothie ever, and it lends itself well to customizing the flavors.

Yield: 1

Preparation Time: 5 minutes

List of Ingredients:

- 2 frozen Bananas
- 1 Peach, peeled and pitted
- 5 frozen Strawberries
- 3 handfuls Baby Spinach or other preferred Greens
- 1 c. Water

MMMMMMMMMMMMMMMMMMMMMMMMMMMMMMMM

Methods:

In a blender, add all Ingredients except for the Greens and pulse a few times. Then add in the Greens and process on high until you have a smooth and creamy texture. Serve.

(33) Melon Lovers Dream Green Smoothie

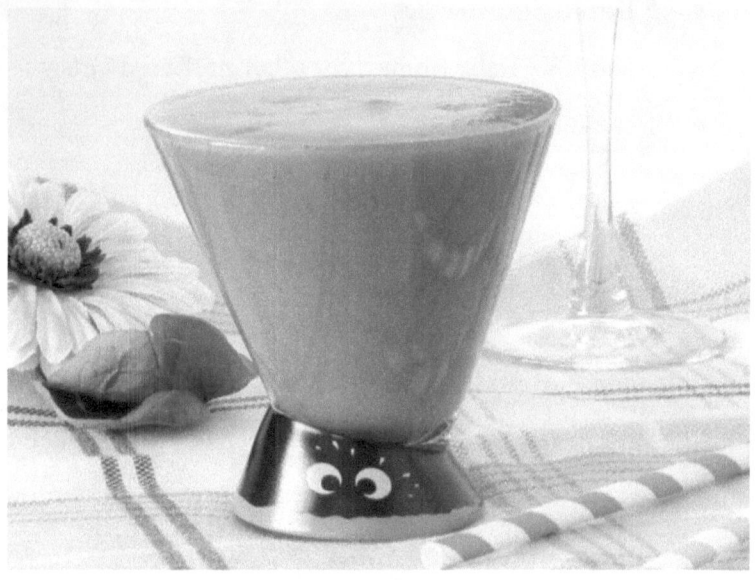

This is a super cleansing smoothie with all the goodness of sweet melons.

Yield: 55 oz.

Preparation Time: 5 minutes

List of Ingredients:

- 2 frozen and peeled Bananas
- 2 c. peeled Cantaloupe, seeded and cubed
- 1 c. seeded Watermelon
- 1 c. seeded and cubed Honeydew Melon
- 3 c. Water
- 5 handfuls greens (your choice)
- ¼ c. Sesame Seeds
- 3 tablespoons Wheat Germ

MMMMMMMMMMMMMMMMMMMMMMMMMMMMMMMMMM

Methods:

In a blender, add all Ingredients except for the greens and pulse a few times. Then add in the Greens and process on high until you have a smooth and creamy texture. Serve.

(34) Wake-Up Green Smoothie

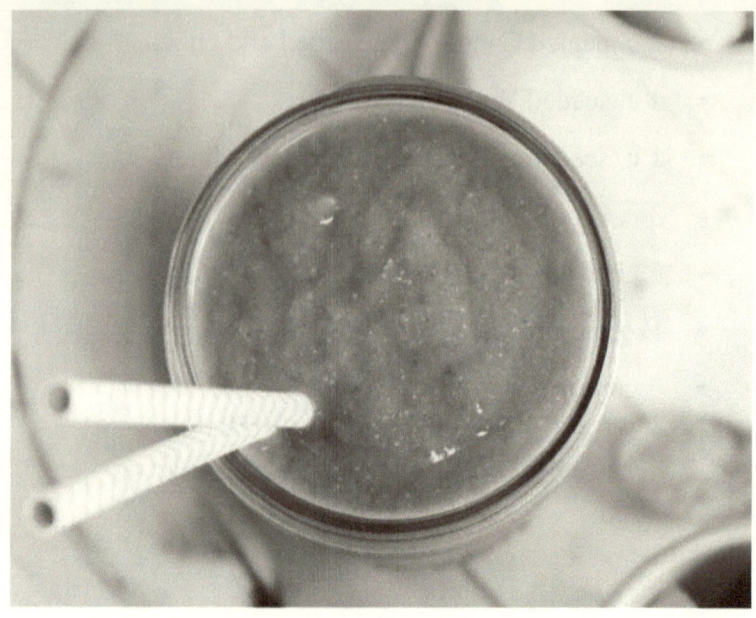

This is an energizing and delicious Green Smoothie, just perfect first thing in the morning.

Yield: 4

Preparation Time: 5 minutes

List of Ingredients:

- 2 frozen Bananas
- 5 Plums, peeled and pitted
- 3 c. Water
- 1 handful Baby Spinach
- 2 handfuls Kale

MMMMMMMMMMMMMMMMMMMMMMMMMMMMMMMMM

Methods:

In a blender, add all Ingredients except for the greens and pulse a few times. Then add in the Greens and process on high until you have a smooth and creamy texture. Serve.

(35) Aloe Parsley Green Smoothie

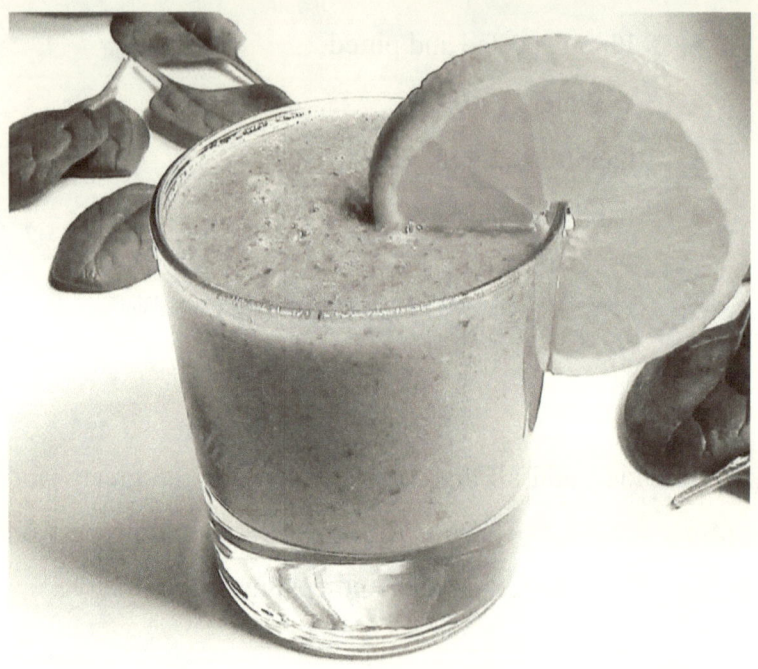

Mildly flavored, yet sweet and fruity; this one is a winner.

Yield: 2

Preparation Time: 5 minutes

List of Ingredients:

- 2 frozen and peeled Bananas
- 1 peeled and seeded Orange
- 1 peeled and cored Apple
- 1 Pear, peeled and cored
- 2 c. Water
- ¼ c. Aloe Vera Juice
- 1 handful Baby Spinach
- 1 handful Bok Choy
- 1 handful Curly Parsley
- 2 tablespoons Flax
- 2 tablespoons Chia Seeds

MMMMMMMMMMMMMMMMMMMMMMMMMMMMMMMM

Methods:

In a blender, add all Ingredients except for the greens and pulse a few times. Then add in the Greens and process on high until you have a smooth and creamy texture. Serve.

(36) Purple Power Breakfast Green Smoothie

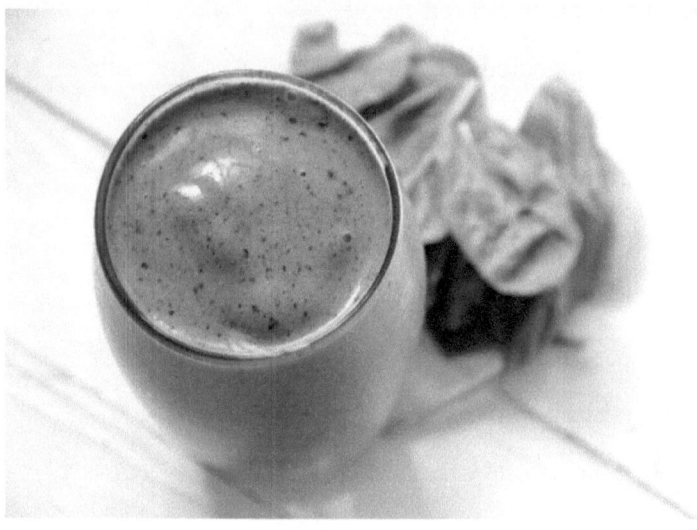

Absolutely delicious and great for breakfast, gives you lots of energy.

Yield: 70 oz.

Preparation Time: 5 minutes

List of Ingredients:

- 1 peeled Apple, cored
- 4 c. fresh Pineapple, peeled and cored
- 1 c. frozen Blueberries
- 3 c. Water
- 1 lb. Baby Spinach or any Green
- 3 tablespoons Flax Seeds

MMMMMMMMMMMMMMMMMMMMMMMMMMMMMMMM

Methods:

In a blender, add all Ingredients except for the greens and pulse a few times. Then add in the Greens and process on high until you have a smooth and creamy texture. Serve.

(37) Energizer Bunny Green Smoothie

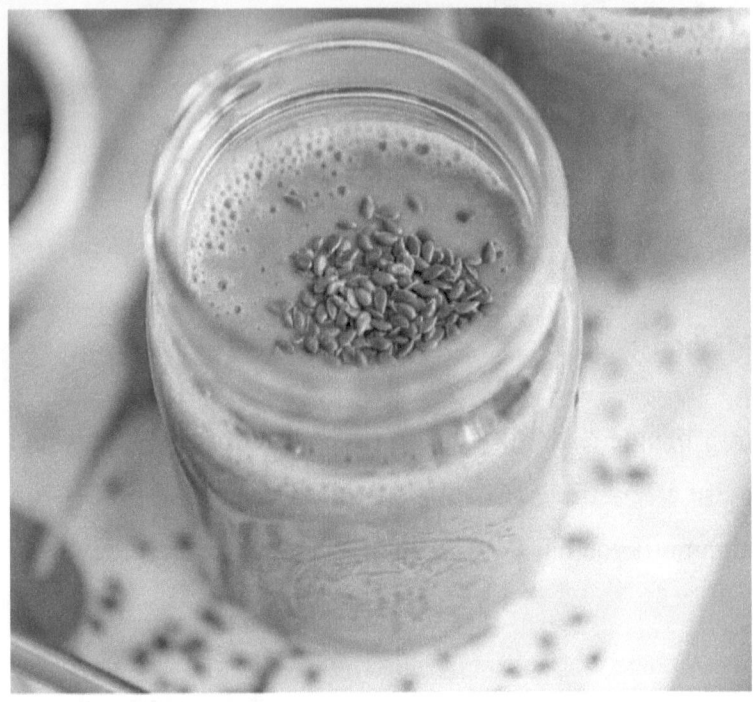

You might find it really hard to be still after this one. Try it before exercise and you'll be amazed how fast the time goes by.

Yield: 40 oz.

Preparation Time: 5 minutes

List of Ingredients:

- 2 frozen and peeled Bananas
- 6 pitted and chopped Dates
- 2 c. Water
- 2 large bunches Dark Green Lettuce
- 2 heaping tablespoons Wheat Germ
- 3 tablespoons Flax Seeds

MMMMMMMMMMMMMMMMMMMMMMMMMMMMMMM

Methods:

In a blender, add all Ingredients except for the greens and pulse a few times. Then add in the Greens and process on high until you have a smooth and creamy texture. Serve.

(38) Mango-Pear Green Smoothie

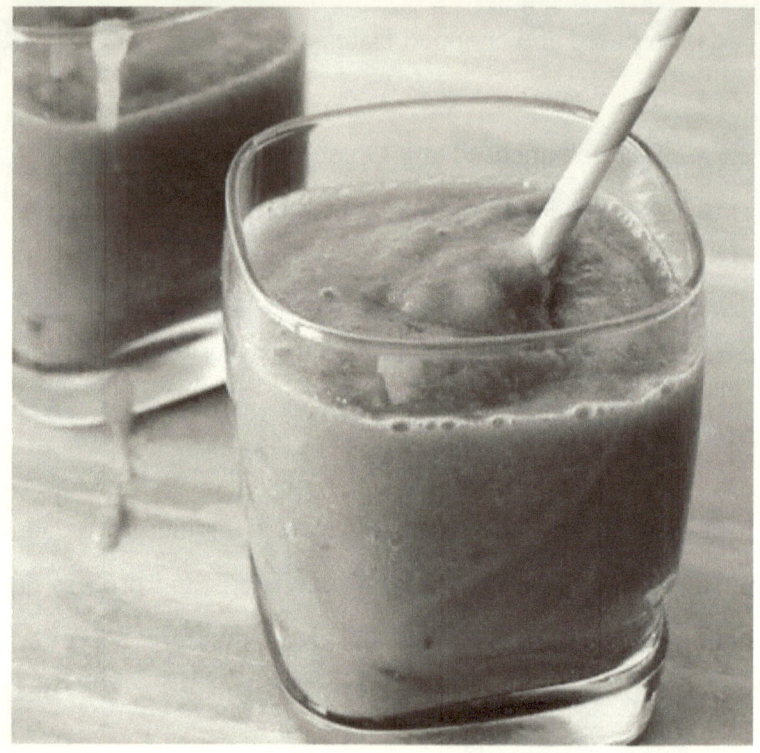

Sweet and tasty, this one is perfect for lunch or snacks.

Yield: 50 oz.

Preparation Time: 5 minutes

List of Ingredients:

- 1 large Mango, peeled and pitted
- 2 Pears, peeled and cored
- 3 c. Water
- 1 handful Purple Kale
- 2-3 handfuls Chard

MMMMMMMMMMMMMMMMMMMMMMMMMMMMMMMMM

Methods:

In a blender, add all Ingredients except for the greens and pulse a few times. Then add in the Greens and process on high until you have a smooth and creamy texture. Serve.

(39) Raspberry Dandelions Green Smoothie

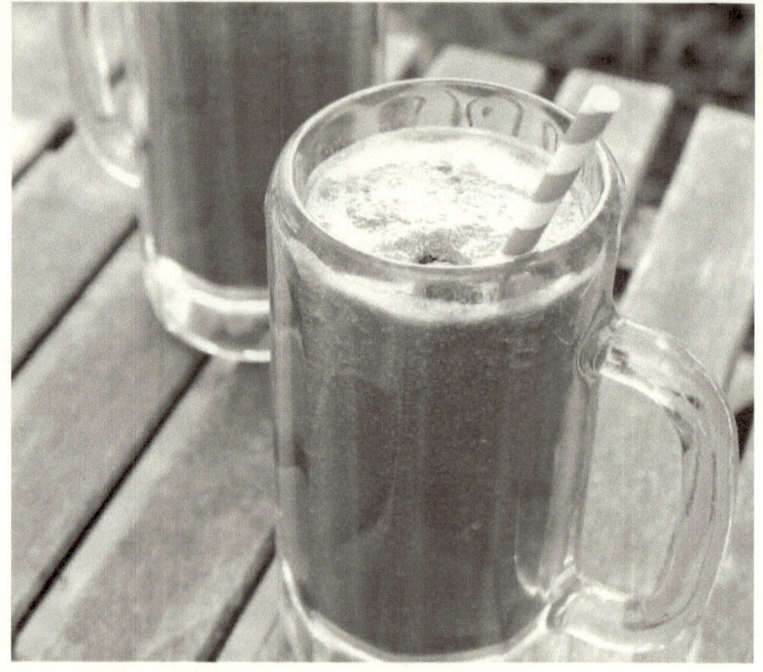

Tart raspberries and dandelion green nutrition is a winning combo.

Yield: 2 – 3

Preparation Time: 5 minutes

List of Ingredients:

- 1 frozen and peeled Banana
- 2 c. frozen Raspberries
- 5 chopped Figs
- 3 c. water
- 1 full bunch Dandelion Greens

MMMMMMMMMMMMMMMMMMMMMMMMMMMMMMMMM

Methods:

In a blender, add all Ingredients except for the greens and pulse a few times. Then add in the Greens and process on high until you have a smooth and creamy texture. Serve.

(40) Strawberry Aloe Vera Green Smoothie

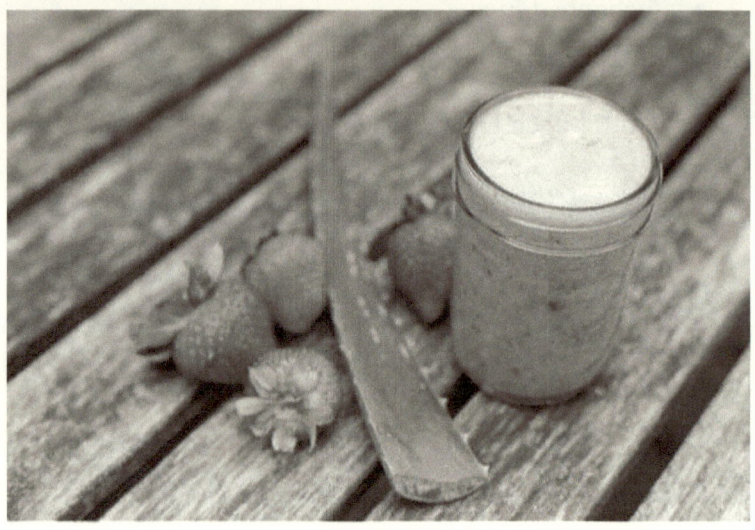

This is a great choice for lunch; light, fresh and fabulous.

Yield: 80 oz.

Preparation Time: 5 minutes

List of Ingredients:

- 4 c. frozen Strawberries
- 2 Pears, peeled and cored
- 3 oz. Aloe Vera Juice
- 3 c. water
- ½ teaspoons Cardamom
- 2 teaspoons Pure Vanilla Extract
- 1 large head Romaine Lettuce (1 lb. or more)

MMMMMMMMMMMMMMMMMMMMMMMMMMMMMMMMM

Methods:

In a blender, add all Ingredients except for the greens and pulse a few times. Then add in the Greens and process on high until you have a smooth and creamy texture. Serve.

(41) Bananalicious Green Smoothie

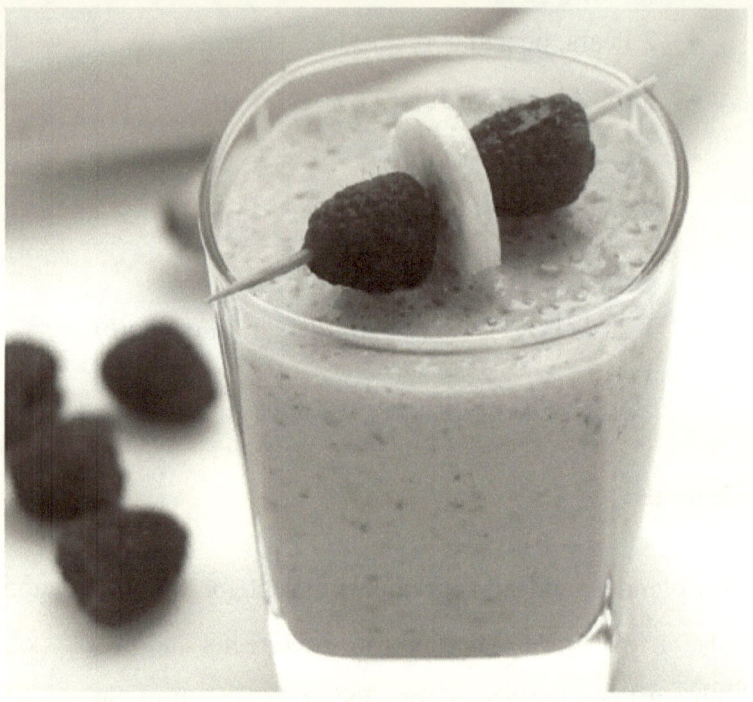

If you love bananas, this is the one for you.

Yield: 60 oz.

Preparation Time: 5 minutes

List of Ingredients:

- 4 frozen and peeled Bananas
- 1 c. frozen Raspberries
- 6 pitted and chopped Dates
- 4 c. Water
- 2 large bunches Dark Green Lettuce
- 3 tablespoons Chia Seeds
- 2 tablespoons Wheat Germ

MMMMMMMMMMMMMMMMMMMMMMMMMMMMMMM

Methods:

In a blender, add all Ingredients except for the greens and pulse a few times. Then add in the Greens and process on high until you have a smooth and creamy texture. Serve.

(42) Orange Beets Green Smoothie

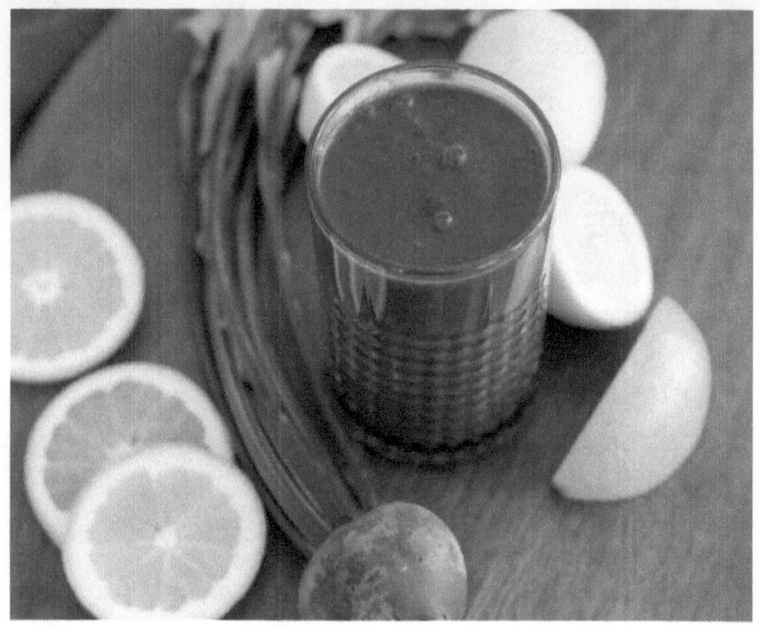

Delightful and different; this one packs an energizing wallop.

Yield: 4

Preparation Time: 5 minutes

List of Ingredients:

- 1 peeled and pitted Ripe Mango
- 3 peeled and seeded Oranges
- ½ c. Aloe Vera Juice
- 3 c. Water
- 2 handfuls Beet Greens with purple stems
- 1 tablespoon Flax Seeds

MMMMMMMMMMMMMMMMMMMMMMMMMMMMMMMM

Methods:

In a blender, add all Ingredients except for the greens and pulse a few times. Then add in the Greens and process on high until you have a smooth and creamy texture. Serve.

(43) Sweet and Tasty Mustard Green Smoothie

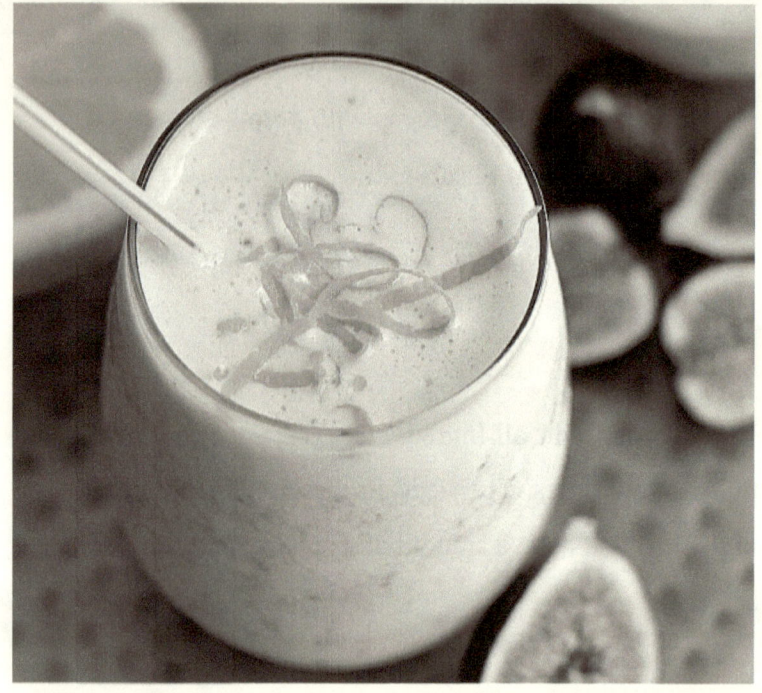

Smoothies are easy to prepare. You will like the flavor of mustard greens and figs.

Yield: 50 oz.

Preparation Time: 5 minutes

List of Ingredients:

- 1 frozen and peeled Banana
- 1 peeled and seeded Orange
- 1 large peeled and cored Fuji Apple
- 6 chopped Figs
- 3 c. water
- 4 handfuls Mustard Greens
- 3 tablespoons Wheat Germ
- 3 tablespoons Flax Seeds

MMMMMMMMMMMMMMMMMMMMMMMMMMMMMMMMM

Methods:

In a blender, add all Ingredients except for the greens and pulse a few times. Then add in the Greens and process on high until you have a smooth and creamy texture. Serve.

(44) My Darling Clementine Green Smoothie

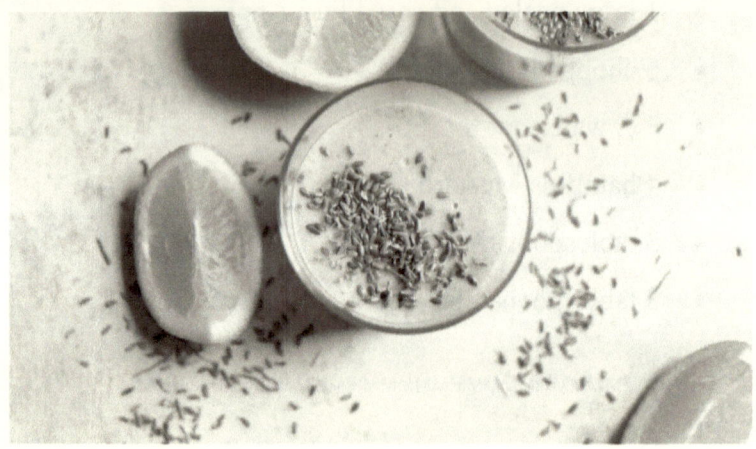

The unusual combination of Clementines and Plums is unbeatable.

Yield: 2

Preparation Time: 5 minutes

List of Ingredients:

- 4 peeled and seeded Clementines
- 2 peeled and pitted Plums
- 1 c. Water or Crushed Ice
- 2 tablespoons Flax Seeds
- 2 tablespoons Chia Seeds
- 4 c. Greens (in accordance to your preference)

MMMMMMMMMMMMMMMMMMMMMMMMMMMMMMMMM

Methods:

In a blender, add all Ingredients except for the greens and pulse a few times. Then add in the Greens and process on high until you have a smooth and creamy texture. Serve.

(45) Green on Green Smoothie

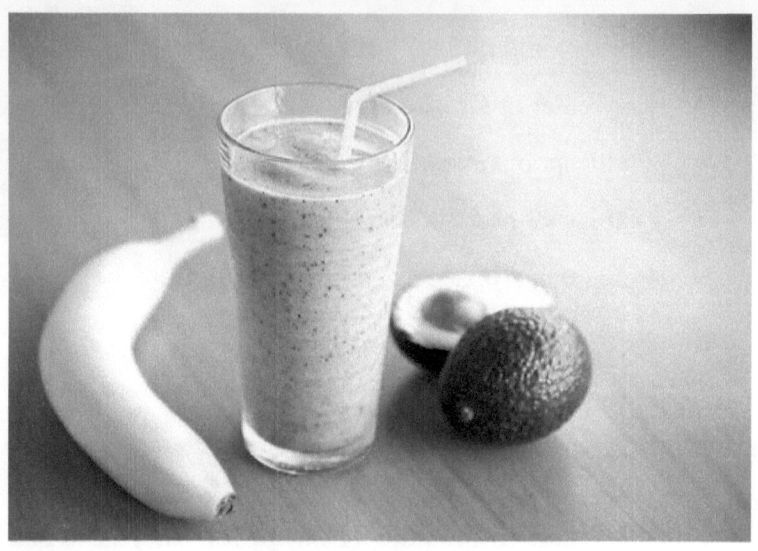

This one is a real fiber and protein miracle that still manages to be tasty.

Yield: 24 oz.

Preparation Time: 5 minutes

List of Ingredients:

- 6 pitted and chopped Dates
- 1 frozen and peeled Banana
- ½ peeled and pitted Avocado
- 3 tablespoons Flax Seeds
- 3 tablespoons Wheat Germ
- 2 c. water
- 2 c. Bok Choy

MMMMMMMMMMMMMMMMMMMMMMMMMMMMMMMM

Methods:

In a blender, add all Ingredients except for the greens and pulse a few times. Then add in the Greens and process on high until you have a smooth and creamy texture. Serve.

(46) Pineapple & Radish Greens Smoothie

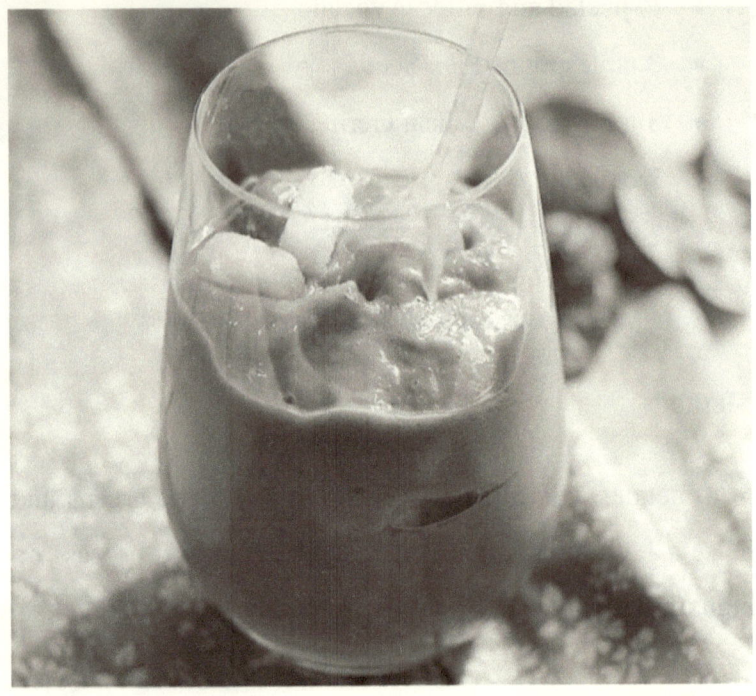

Did you know that the greens of the radish were a great option and chock full of nutrition?

Yield: 64 oz.

Preparation Time: 5 minutes

List of Ingredients:

- 2 frozen Bananas, peeled
- 1 peeled and pitted ripe Mango
- ½ peeled and cored ripe Pineapple
- 3 c. Water or Crushed Ice
- 3 handfuls Radish Greens
- ½ c. Goji Berries
- 3 tablespoons Flax Seeds
- 2 tablespoons Wheat Germ

MMMMMMMMMMMMMMMMMMMMMMMMMMMMMMMM

Methods:

In a blender, add all Ingredients except for the greens and pulse a few times. Then add in the Greens and process on high until you have a smooth and creamy texture. Serve.

(47) Raspy Orange Green Smoothie

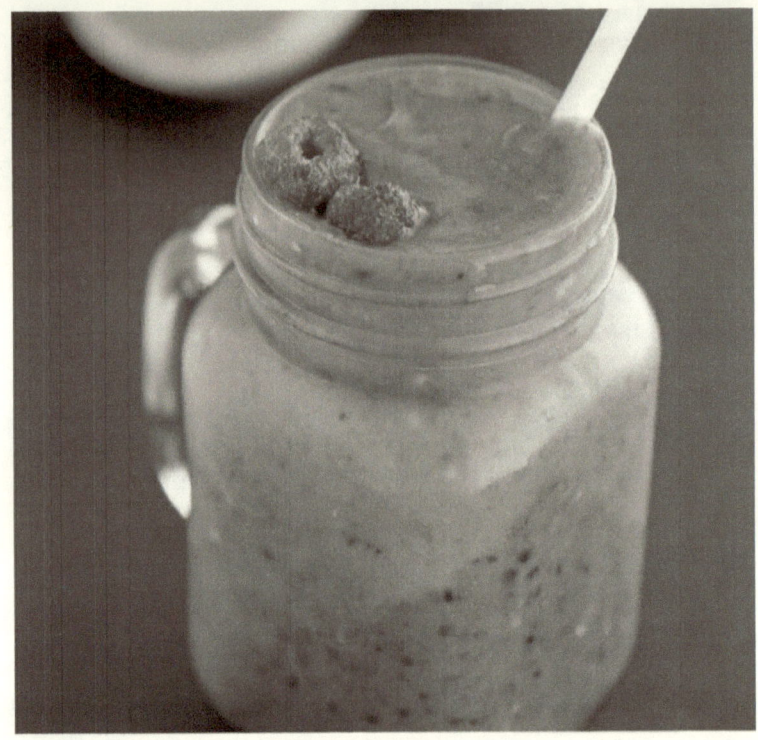

A little different and a whole lot tasty.

Yield: 36 oz.

Preparation Time: 5 minutes

List of Ingredients:

- 2 peeled and seeded Oranges
- 2 c. fresh or frozen Raspberries
- 8 pitted and chopped Dates
- 1 tablespoon Chia Seeds
- 2 c. Water
- 5 handfuls Lambs quarters or your preferred greens

MMMMMMMMMMMMMMMMMMMMMMMMMMMMMMMM

Methods:

In a blender, add all Ingredients except for the greens and pulse a few times. Then add in the Greens and process on high until you have a smooth and creamy texture. Serve.

(48) Orange Goji Green Smoothie

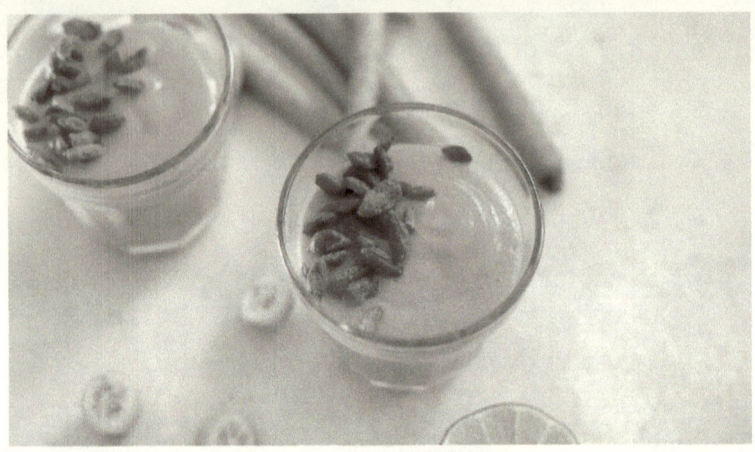

This is a superb recipe that will include the taste of Goji berries. You will love it and is easy to prepare.

Yield: 20 oz.

Preparation Time: 5 minutes

List of Ingredients:

- 1 Orange, peeled and seeded
- 2 Dates, pitted and chopped
- 3 tablespoons Goji Berries
- 1 c. Water or Crushed Ice
- 3 c. Mixed Dark Greens (or your preferred choice)
- 1 tablespoon Wheat Germ

MMMMMMMMMMMMMMMMMMMMMMMMMMMMMMMMM

Methods:

In a blender, add all Ingredients except for the greens and pulse a few times. Then add in the Greens and process on high until you have a smooth and creamy texture. Serve.

(49) Plum Bananas Green Smoothie

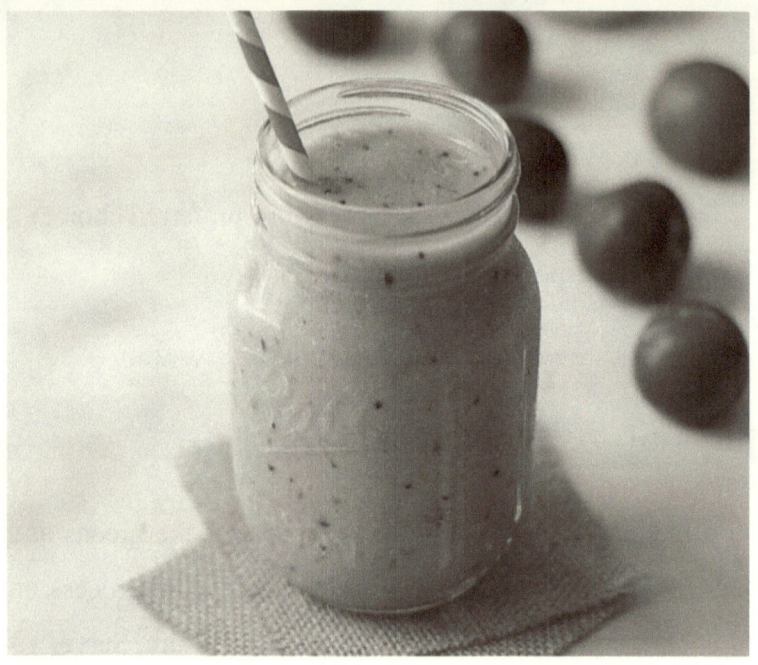

You will go "plum bananas" over this taste bud titillating treat.

Yield: 64 oz.

Preparation Time: 5 minutes

List of Ingredients:

- 4 peeled and pitted Plums
- 2 frozen and peeled Bananas
- 2 peeled and seeded Oranges
- 4 chopped Dates
- 3 c. Water
- 4 handfuls Bok Choy
- 3 tablespoons Flax Seeds
- 3 tablespoons Goji Berries

MMMMMMMMMMMMMMMMMMMMMMMMMMMMMMM

Methods:

In a blender, add all Ingredients except for the greens and pulse a few times. Then add in the Greens and process on high until you have a smooth and creamy texture. Serve.

(50) Orange Cream Green Smoothie Snack

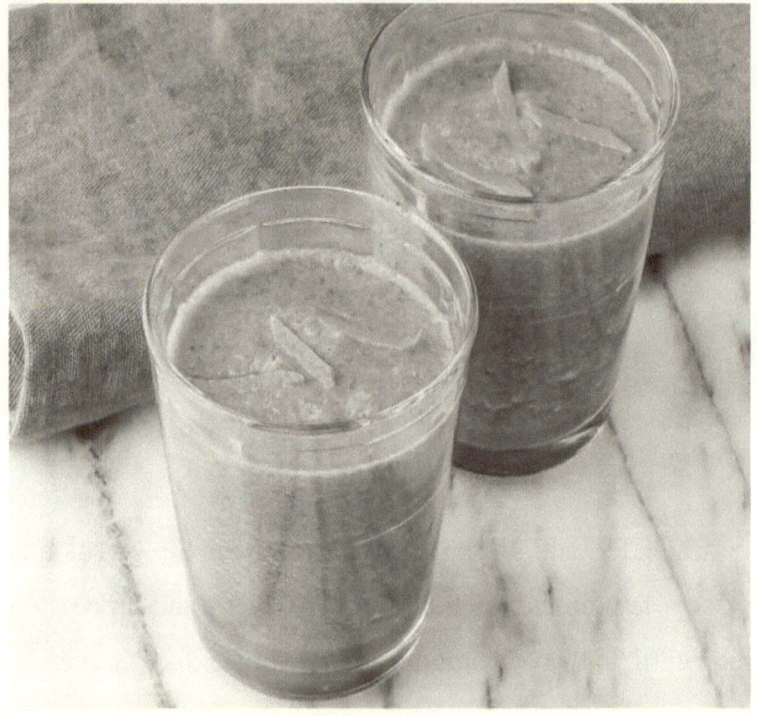

This one is a fabulous choice for your snack times; you'll think you've had ice cream.

Yield: 1

Preparation Time: 5 minutes

List of Ingredients:

- 1 peeled and seeded Orange
- ¼ peeled and pitted Avocado
- 1 c. Nut Milk or Coconut Water
- 1 handful Romaine Lettuce
- 1 handful Baby Spinach
- ½ teaspoons Pure Vanilla Extract
- Sweetener if preferred

MMMMMMMMMMMMMMMMMMMMMMMMMMMMMMMM

Methods:

In a blender, add all Ingredients except for the greens and pulse a few times. Then add in the Greens and process on high until you have a smooth and creamy texture. Serve.

About the Author

A native of Indianapolis, Indiana, Valeria Ray found her passion for cooking while she was studying English Literature at Oakland City University. She decided to try a cooking course with her friends and the experience changed her forever. She enrolled at the Art Institute of Indiana which offered extensive courses in the culinary Arts. Once Ray dipped her toe in the cooking world, she never looked back.

When Valeria graduated, she worked in French restaurants in the Indianapolis area until she became the head chef at one of the 5-star establishments in the area. Valeria's attention to taste and visual detail caught the eye of a local business person who expressed an interest in publishing her recipes. Valeria began her secondary career authoring cookbooks and e-books which she tackled with as much talent and gusto as her first career. Her passion for food leaps off the page of her books which have colourful anecdotes and stunning pictures of dishes she has prepared herself.

Valeria Ray lives in Indianapolis with her husband of 15 years, Tom, her daughter, Isobel and their loveable Golden Retriever, Goldy. Valeria enjoys cooking special dishes in her large, comfortable kitchen where the family gets involved in preparing meals. This successful, dynamic chef is an inspiration to culinary students and novice cooks everywhere.

••••••••••••••••••••

Author's Afterthoughts

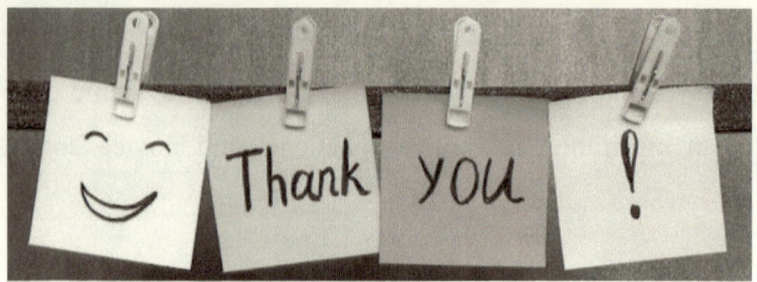

Thank you for Purchasing my book and taking the time to read it from front to back. I am always grateful when a reader chooses my work and I hope you enjoyed it!

With the vast selection available online, I am touched that you chose to be purchasing my work and take valuable time out of your life to read it. My hope is that you feel you made the right decision.

I very much would like to know what you thought of the book. Please take the time to write an honest and informative review on Amazon.com. Your experience and opinions will be of great benefit to me and those readers looking to make an informed choice.

With much thanks,

Valeria Ray